The indomitable lady doctors

Carlotta Hacker

Clarke, Irwin & Company Limited
Toronto/Vancouver

A project of the
Federation of Medical Women of Canada
C.M.A. House, P.O. Box 8244, Ottawa K1G 3H7

Financial assistance provided by
the physicians of Ontario through
The Physicians' Services Incorporated Foundation
and by physicians across Canada who made personal donations
through The Federation of Medical Women of Canada

PREFACE

THIS book is the Golden Jubilee project of the Federation of Medical Women of Canada. The heroines are real, and it was because of the need to put on record the accomplishment of this group of Canadian women that the project was undertaken. Through their stories our history comes alive in an interesting and exciting way.

We were indeed fortunate to find a professional such as Carlotta Hacker who could both research the subject and write with colour and charm. The information in these pages has been well researched; Carlotta Hacker travelled from coast to coast in search of facts and, from the wealth of material, chose the heroines of this book. All who read may not find their favourite "lady doctor," but if you have known one I am sure you will enjoy the tales of the others, stories that will delight not only doctors but people in all walks of life, young and old, women and men.

The Indomitable Lady Doctors is a memorial to pioneering women in Canadian medicine. It will help to keep alive their spirit of devotion and dedication. It will, we hope, challenge all women to realize that there is no easy way to achieve the excellence that must be attained if we are to continue to give dedicated service.

EVA MADER MACDONALD, M.D., C.M.
Chairman of the Jubilee Book Committee,
Federation of Medical Women of Canada

Toronto
May, 1974

ACKNOWLEDGEMENTS

FIRST of all, I should like to thank the Federation of Medical Women of Canada for asking me to research and write this book, and in particular I wish to thank Dr Eva Mader Macdonald, who has been the moving spirit behind the project and whose enthusiasm and involvement has been of the greatest assistance and encouragement.

Secondly, I am indebted to the many archivists and librarians who have assisted me in the search for material. It is not possible to mention them all individually, but I do want to stress how extremely grateful I am for the specialized and very willing help I have been given in libraries right across Canada.

More specifically, I am grateful to Isobel Rae, both for the information she sent me about Dr Barry and for the use of material from her book *The Strange Story of Dr James Barry;* to Major-General T.W. Carrick, Commandant and Dean of the Royal Army Medical College, Millbank, London, and to Admiral Richard Roberts, the Surgeon General, Canadian Forces, for the help they gave me in the research on Dr Barry. I am also very grateful to Joan St George Saunders for the invaluable research she did in London on Dr Barry and on the other women doctors who had connections with Great Britain.

Mr Hudson J. Stowe and Miss Hilda I. Stowe have been most helpful in providing me with information on Dr Emily Stowe and Dr Augusta Stowe-Gullen. I also wish to express my thanks to the Archives of Wilfrid Laurier University, Waterloo, for granting me permission to quote from the Stowe Scrapbooks; and the Archives of Victoria University, the University of Toronto, Toronto Western Hospital, and the Public Archives of Canada for making available to me their material on members of the Stowe family.

Mr James Anderson, Perth County Archivist, has been of great assistance in the research on Dr Jennie Trout and I am extremely thankful for all the help he has given me. I am indebted to Pauline Johnston, Associate Medical Librarian, Medical College of Pennsylvania, for the material she sent on Dr Trout and the other graduates from the the Woman's Medical College of Pennsylvania.

I wish to extend my thanks to the Queen's University Archives, Kingston, Ontario, for giving me permission to quote from their material, and to say how grateful I am to the staffs of the Archives and of the Lorne Pierce Collection at Queen's for the help I received when researching material on Dr Elizabeth Smith-Shortt and the other Queen's graduates.

Dr Enid Johnson MacLeod has been of the greatest assistance in providing me with information on Maritimers as well as on many other women doctors; I also want to thank the staff of the Public Archives of Nova Scotia.

I am grateful to Mrs E.A. Backman for the information she gave me about her grandmother, Dr Charlotte Ross, and to Miss Carol Whitfield, Historian, Department of Indian Affairs and Northern Development, for making available to me the results of her research on Dr Ross. The Provincial Archives of Manitoba were most helpful in supplying material on Dr Ross as well as on Dr Yeomans. Miss Edith Paterson of the *Winnipeg Free Press* kindly provided me with information on Dr Yeomans and I wish to thank her for offering me the results of her research.

The United Church Archives, the Archives of the Anglican Church of Canada and the Library of Emmanual College, Victoria University, have all given me the greatest assistance in my search for information on medical missionaries. I also wish to thank Dr A.L. Chute and Miss L. Chute for telling me the background story of their mother, Dr Pearl Chute.

For material on Dr Elizabeth Matheson and on her contemporaries in the West I am indebted to her daughter, Mrs Ruth Matheson Buck; I also wish to thank Professor Audrey M. Kerr, Medical Librarian, University of Manitoba, for the information she provided on Manitoba graduates.

Acknowledgements

I am grateful to Dr H.E. MacDermot for permission to quote from his book *Maude Abbott; a Memoir;* to Dr E.H. Bensley, Department of the History of Medicine at McGill University, for the help he has given me with matters relating to Bishop's Medical College and McGill University; and to the Osler Library and the Department of the History of Medicine at McGill. I also extend my thanks to Dr de la Broquerie Fortier, Dr Edouard Desjardins and Dr Jacques Abourbih for their assistance with the research on early medical women in the Province of Quebec.

I wish to thank Dr Mary Lee Edward for allowing me to quote from her war diary, and to use material from her Memoir; Mrs Joan Fellows and Mr Peter Leacock for giving me so much information about their mother, Dr Evelyn Windsor Leacock; and the Glenbow-Alberta Institute for making available to me material on Dr Windsor Leacock and other women doctors of Alberta. I am grateful to S/Sgt Major J. Robinson for telling me about his work with Dr Frances McGill, and to the Royal Canadian Mounted Police, both in Ottawa and Regina, for the material they provided on Dr Frances McGill.

Finally, I wish to thank the Canadian Medical Association, the Royal College of Physicians and Surgeons of Canada, and the many physicians, medical librarians and university staffs, in the United States as well as in Canada, who have so patiently assisted me in the search for information about our early women doctors.

CONTENTS

LIST OF ILLUSTRATIONS & ACKNOWLEDGEMENTS

JAMES MIRANDA STUART BARRY
Royal Army Medical College, Millbank, London

EMILY STOWE
Patricia Emily Stowe, great-great granddaughter of Emily Stowe

AUGUSTA STOWE-GULLEN
From A History of Victoria University, *by C. B. Sissons, University of Toronto Press, 1952*

JENNIE TROUT
Queen's University Archives

ELIZABETH SMITH-SHORTT
Queen's University Archives

ELIZABETH BEATTY
Queen's University Archives

ALICE MCGILLIVRAY
Queen's University Archives

CHARLOTTE ROSS
Mrs E.A. Backman

AMELIA YEOMANS
Miss Muriel Sissons

SUSIE RIJNHART
Emmanuel College Library

PEARL CHUTE
Miss L. Chute

ELIZABETH MATHESON
    Mrs Ruth Matheson Buck
CLASS PHOTO
    Mrs Ruth Matheson Buck
MAUDE ABBOTT
    Dr H.E. MacDermot
IRMA LEVASSEUR
    L'Hôpital Sainte-Justine
MARY LEE EDWARD
    Dr Mary Lee Edward
EVELYN WINDSOR
    Mrs Joan Fellows
FRANCES MCGILL
    RCMP Quarterly *and Mr and Mrs E.R. McGill*
MARY PERCY JACKSON
    Dr Mary Percy Jackson & Glenbow-Alberta Institute
MODERN
    Dr Eva Mader Macdonald
ONTARIO MEDICAL COLLEGE FOR WOMEN *(back cover)*
    Women's College Hospital

The indomitable lady doctors

1

The eccentric Dr Barry

THE FIRST woman doctor to practise medicine in Canada was a man
— according to her death certificate, which firmly says 'male'. He/
she was Dr James Miranda Stuart Barry,[1] the British Army medical
officer who, in 1857, was appointed Inspector-General of Hospitals
for both Upper and Lower Canada. In other words, Barry was made
head of the whole works, chief military doctor in Canada, and
supervisor of hospitals in Kingston, Montreal, Quebec and Toronto.

By the time Dr Barry arrived in Canada to take up this exalted
position, she had successfully posed as a man for more than forty
years. During those years she had gained the reputation of being a
highly competent doctor, an outstanding surgeon, a rather quirky
dietician, a difficult associate, an uncongenial member of the mess-
room — she wouldn't get drunk and tell dirty stories — and a hot-
tempered redhead who was quick to take offence, and might even
fight a duel to defend her honour. With good reason she was considered an eccentric — but a brilliant one. And although many
people found her hilariously effeminate, very few suspected that
she might simply be feminine. It was only after she died that her
secret was discovered when she was laid out for burial and seen to
have the body of a woman. As a result of this disclosure, Dr Barry
died as she had lived — the centre of a raging controversy.[2]

Throughout her life, Dr Barry was continually embroiled in disputes, for she had a blind spot, a lack of political acumen, that

caused her to follow what she plainly saw as her duty and write any amount of outspoken letters to the Army Medical Department, regardless and apparently oblivious of the fact that she had a formidable body of superiors ranged against her. For instance, in her first overseas posting, to Cape Town, she was doing extremely well until she crossed swords with the authorities. She had arrived in Cape Town in 1816 with a good Edinburgh degree and three untroubled years of army service behind her. As she had also arrived with some letters of introduction to the Governor, her future looked most promising.

And all went well at first. She performed her duties so meticulously that she was promoted from Assistant Surgeon to Colonial Medical Inspector and Physician to the Governor's Household. She became a close friend of the Governor — such a close friend as to cause gossip. She probably saved his life when he caught typhus fever. In addition, she made a name for herself as a surgeon by performing one of the first Caesarean operations in which both mother and child survived.

Dr Barry must have been very pleased with her progress. She was moving steadily onwards and upwards, and so were her reputation and salary. And she was acting the male part so convincingly that she had been universally accepted as a man, if rather an odd one, for she tended to overact her part, strutting rather than walking, and trying to be aggressively male. This caused comment because it didn't match her appearance. She was only five feet tall, a slim rather fragile figure, with smooth cheeks, large eyes and small hands and feet. Her only masculine feature was an unusually long nose, and that just made her look peculiar.

Lord Albemarle met her around this time, and later wrote a description that shows she was already attracting a good deal of notice:

There was at this time at the Cape a person whose eccentricities attracted universal attention — Dr James Barry, staff-surgeon to the garrison, and the Governor's medical adviser. . . . I had heard so much of this capricious, yet privileged gentleman, that I had a great curiosity to see him. I shortly afterwards sat next him at dinner at one of the regimental messes. In this learned Pundit I beheld a beardless lad, apparently of my own age, with an unmistakably Scotch type of countenance — reddish hair, high cheek bones. There was a certain effeminacy in his manner, which he seemed to be always striving to overcome. His style of conversation was greatly superior to that one usually heard at a mess-table in those days of *non*-competitive examination.[3]

Many people must have been as curious as Lord Albemarle, and of course a great many ribald comments were made. But most of them were made out of hearing, for Barry was quick to take offence and had already fought a duel because of a personal remark. One had to be wary of this peppery little doctor.

Unfortunately, the peppery little doctor wasn't as wary as her associates. Her troubles began — or, rather, she began her troubles — almost as soon as she felt secure, and it was not long before she was fighting a pitched battle against the authorities because she refused to license an apothecary who had plenty of experience but no qualifications. When the ruling was made against Dr Barry, she refused to accept it — which put her friend the Governor in an awkward position. She then moved blithely on to make life even more uncomfortable for him by criticising conditions in the Leper Institution.

The lepers, she said, were not being looked after properly. They should be better fed, given mutton at least once a day, fresh vegetables, milk and rice. They should bath at least twice a week, their bedding should be changed frequently and 'no *cruelty* nor deprivation of food must ever be resorted to.'[4]

Rather than agree to these reforms, the manager of the Leper Institution threatened to resign. But Dr Barry did win some of her points.

She won some points in her next battle too, which was over conditions in the jail and the lunatic asylum, but she went into the attack with her habitual lack of caution, gained too many enemies, and found herself without a job. She wasn't exactly dismissed, but the ground was removed from under her. The office of Colonial Medical Inspector was abolished, and Dr Barry discovered that if she wished to continue to work in Cape Town she could only do so as a junior member of a committee staffed by her antagonists. This she refused to do, and after a humiliating few months she was glad to leave the country she had become so fond of, and accept a posting to Mauritius as Staff-Surgeon.

From then on, Dr Barry's career followed the pattern she had set in the Cape: outstanding and dedicated work, successful reforms, improved conditions and more nourishing and palatable food for both troops and prisoners, acrimonious disputes with the authorities ... followed by a worrying few months on half-pay and too many incautious letters to the War Office and Army Medical Department.

On one occasion Dr Barry was actually arrested for her behaviour and sent home under guard. But when she arrived in England, she was reprieved. Although she left almost every country under a cloud of disfavour, she always seemed to get pardonned — and promoted. It has been hinted that this was because she had a bevy of powerful, aristocratic friends, lurking just out of sight but ready to support her when the need arose. She did indeed have a few influential friends. At one time she called on Lord Raglan to defend her actions, but he had his own problems just then, trying to cope with the Crimean War, so she didn't get much help there. But undoubtedly she did occasionally receive help from high places. All the same, one can't put her success down to her string-pulling. She did pull strings and she was very ambitious, but she was also an extremely competent doctor. The Army Medical Department appreciated this. They knew she was difficult — how they knew! — but they also knew that she was one of the top 'men' in the field.

And so Dr Barry received promotion after promotion, and travelled round the Empire and prospective Empire leaving a trail of reforms and enemies behind her. From Mauritius she was posted to Jamaica, where she saw her first active service during the 'Negroes Insurrection', from Jamaica she went to St Helena, from St Helena to Trinidad, from Trinidad to Malta ... to Corfu ... to the Crimea (on active leave!) ... and, eventually, to Canada.[5]

Dr Barry was in her sixties when she arrived in Canada to take up the position of Inspector-General of Hospitals. She no longer looked like a young boy, but she was still very small and slight, and her nose seemed longer than ever. So did her sword, which somehow managed to look larger and clumsier as she grew older, so that she clanked along, with the sword almost touching the ground. Dr Barry had always enjoyed her accoutrements and uniforms. She liked to present a dapper appearance with her cocked hats and plumes and imposing epaulettes, but she had never before had much of a chance to wear furs. Now she went all out and wrapped herself in musk-ox fur as she drove round Montreal in a bright

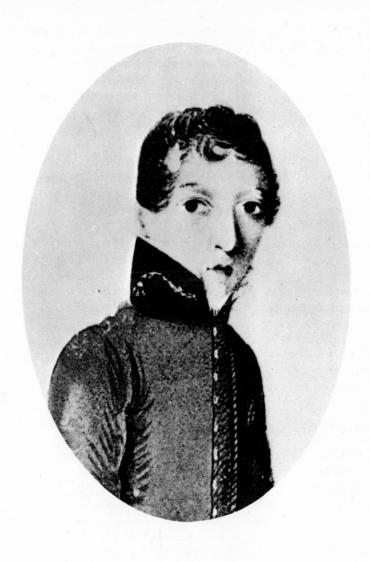

Dr James Barry in uniform

red sleigh. It was almost as if she was trying to call attention to herself.

For some years she had been accompanied almost everywhere by a large black manservant and a small white dog — and, as if this wasn't enough to make everyone stare, she now added a uniformed footman and coachman to her entourage, as she drove round the city in her magnificent red sleigh with its silver bells. Canada must have wondered what on earth Britain had sent this time.

Britain had sent a reformer, as everyone soon discovered. The first matter to receive attention was the troops' diet. By this time Dr Barry had become a vegetarian, living mainly on fruit, vegetables and milk, but she did appreciate that the men required a more substantial diet. She found that they were getting it — one pound of beef and one pound of bread a day — but she considered the food dull. Soon she was issuing streams of recommendations and instructions, saying that the men should have mutton and salt pork as well as beef, and that the kitchens should be provided with ovens so that the troops could have 'the cheering change of a roast instead of eternal boiled beef and soup.'[6]

Having dealt with diet, her first priority, she was soon suggesting — or ordering — alterations in the Quebec barracks, insisting that both sewage and drainage were inadequate and that pipes should be installed so that water didn't have to be delivered by cart. She also found the hospitals inadequate. They were overcrowded, and both pillows and mattresses were made of straw. So bring in hair mattresses and feather pillows!

If Dr Barry ran up another list of enemies in the administrative departments, she must certainly have been well liked by the troops.

Her most startling discovery in Canada was in the married quarters, or in the lack of them, for no facilities were provided for the ordinary soldier. If a man had a wife, she slept in his bed in the barracks. It was natural that Dr Barry should find this far more shocking than the previous Inspector-General had done, and she quickly set about getting the situation altered, recommending a private room for each family. Present conditions encouraged drunkenness, she said. Obviously an innocent young bride would resort to drink, and then to crime and depravity, if she was forced to live in such a rough manner.

All these reforms seem obvious in the twentieth century and

they seemed obvious to Dr Barry too. After all, this was the great age of hospital reform when Florence Nightingale was carrying out far more drastic measures. But Florence Nightingale was not as tactless as Dr Barry — nor so uncivil apparently. When the two reformers met in the Crimea, Miss Nightingale was obliged to stand in the sun while Dr Barry, seated haughtily on horseback, delivered a public reprimand. Florence Nightingale was furious:

(He) kept me standing in the midst of quite a crowd of soldiers, commissariat servants, camp followers etc. etc. every one of whom behaved like a gentleman, during the scolding I received, while (she) behaved like a brute. After (she) was dead, I was told (he) was a woman. I should say (she) was the most hardened creature I ever met.[7]

'(He) - (She)' certainly didn't exercise much tact on that occasion, though one has to allow for the fact that Florence Nightingale wasn't an easy character either. But she did gather supporters easily — a gift that Dr Barry lacked. Although Dr Barry made a few good friends during her life, most of her colleagues disliked her. They found her too autocratic. And too odd. This had the unfortunate result that their evidence about Dr Barry, after her death, is laced with sneers and innuendos, and instead of describing a most remarkable woman doctor, they describe a petty little crank, who was thoroughly unreliable and only tolerably good at 'his' job.

In Canada, Dr Barry proved herself extremely good at her job, as she had so often done before. Moreover, it was a very responsible job, one of the most senior positions in the medical services. But this was to be her last posting. She became ill in Canada. First of all she suffered from bronchitis, and then, in 1859, she went down with influenza and became so ill that she was sent back to England.

She must have dreaded illness more than most people, for it was the obvious occasion for her sex to be discovered. It had, in fact, been discovered in Trinidad when she was ill with yellow fever. Believing herself to be dying, she had requested that she should be buried with her clothes on. As it turned out, this precaution would have been useless, for her assistant surgeon had visited her — strictly against orders — to see if he could do anything for her, and on stripping back the bedclothes, had seen to his amazement that Dr Barry looked like a woman. Fortunately, Dr Barry recovered consciousness at that moment and groggily swore the assistant surgeon and another witness to secrecy. Both men kept their word — until the Great Revelation was made in 1865.

In the meantime, Dr Barry found herself leaving Canada, far from well, to face an Army Medical Board in England. She could cope with that, she had already coped with plenty of medical boards, but she couldn't cope with the findings of this one. They declared her unfit for further service.

She certainly wasn't fit. Already weak from influenza, she had had a very rough journey from Canada — some stories say that she was even shipwrecked — and she had had to spend some days recuperating in Liverpool before she was strong enough to travel to London. In any case, she was about sixty-five by now, so the Board's ruling made sense. But, of course, Dr Barry wouldn't accept this. She said the Medical Board was made up of very *junior* officers, and she began her retirement by contesting their decision and writing a long letter to the Secretary of State for War, asking to be returned to Canada, or sent somewhere else — and virtually asking for a knighthood:

I am now prepared to serve Her Majesty in any quarter of the Globe to which I may be sent [she wrote], and am loath to close a career which impartially may be deemed to have been a useful and faithful one without some special mark of Her Majesty's gracious favor.[8]

Dr Barry didn't get the knighthood, nor was she sent back to Canada. And when she died six years later, she didn't even manage to keep her secret. As she had feared, it became the gossip of the day.

Even now, nearly two hundred years after she was born, Dr Barry's story is still the subject of argument, if not gossip, for it gives rise to so many questions. Who was she really? How on earth did a girl, born in the 1790's, manage, in the first place, to get so well educated as to be accepted by Edinburgh University? How did she manage to keep her sex a secret for so many years — and what was her sex? Was she truly female? Some people think she was a hermaphrodite.

It is, at least, fairly simple to explain how Dr Barry kept her secret. She lived a rather secluded life, protected by a large black servant and a dog, she never shared accommodation if she could avoid it, and when forced to share a cabin, for instance, wouldn't undress until her roommate had left. She was therefore thought to be extraordinarily modest, and this reputation must have been useful when, from time to time, she was subjected to a medical examination.

The other questions are not so easy to answer, partly because Dr Barry intentionally gave false accounts of her origins, and partly because so much mystery surrounds her that the literature on her contains as much fiction as fact. One story has her serving so gallantly at Waterloo that she received instant promotion. But the Army records show that she was in England during 1815.

Fortunately, the records of her life as James Barry are well documented, and they go back to her acceptance by Edinburgh University in 1809 and her graduation in 1812. She was apparently a very eager student, took far more courses than were required, and went on from Edinburgh to study surgery under Sir Astley Cooper in London. Since Sir Astley Cooper was breaking new ground in the field of surgery, since Edinburgh was famed for its medical school, and since young Barry was an abnormally industrious student, one can see how she became such an outstanding physician. Canada's first woman doctor was certainly of very high calibre.

But the early records do more than explain how Barry became such an exceptional doctor. Every now and again one gets a clue as to how it all happened in the first place, and what she was up to during what might be called her feminine years, for the records show that she was the protegée, and probably the niece, of a man called James Barry, a member of the Royal Academy of Arts. This is significant because, when one looks at Barry-artist and his friends, one can see how his protegée found the opportunity to educate herself.

Barry-artist was a witty and sparkling character, an Irishman by birth, who had been hailed as a prodigy in his youth, had travelled round Europe, settled in London, and had held the position of Professor of Painting at the Royal Academy until he was expelled for publicly criticising his associates.[9] Widely educated himself, he was a firm believer in education, and a friend of such people as Edmund Burke, Dr Johnson and Dr Burney. Most significantly, he was also a follower of Mary Wollstonecraft, who wrote *Vindication of the Rights of Woman*. A young girl brought up in this atmosphere could hardly have avoided acquiring a most stimulating education, spurred on as she was by her free-thinking relative to question as well as to learn. Unfortunately, Barry-artist died before his protegée went up to Edinburgh, but this fact is also significant. It explains why she chose that particular name as her alias.

Three other characters can be traced to the feminine years, and they all play their part in unravelling the mystery. One was a woman called Mrs Bulkeley, who chaperoned the young student during her first year in Edinburgh. The second was a man called Dr Fryer — *doctor* Fryer. And the third was a man called General Francisco de Miranda, who was a family friend, another formative influence, and whose name also appears in Barry's alias — James Miranda Barry. Like the artist, General Miranda believed very strongly in the importance of education. He is said to have owned the best private library in London, which included a complete mini-library of medical books; and the young medical student was given the run of this library. How she managed to get educated is therefore not so very puzzling.

Who she was will always remain a slight puzzle, but it seems probable that she was the daughter of Mrs Bulkeley, the woman who accompanied her to Edinburgh. A Miss Bulkeley wrote a commemorative poem to Barry-artist when he died, and even more suggestive is a letter that young James Barry wrote to General Miranda.[10] In the postscript she reminds the General that nobody at Edinburgh knows anything about Mrs Bulkeley's daughter, and she begs both him and Dr Fryer to be very careful about what they write in their letters.

Whether she really was a *she* will always remain open to speculation, since Dr Barry was buried before the story of her sex became public, so no post-mortem was made. The most acceptable explanation at the time was that she was a male hermaphrodite — for of course it was impossible that any female could have achieved as much as Dr Barry had done. There is still a body of opinion that goes along with this explanation, but it is worth noting that the theory is based almost entirely on three very strong prejudices: anti-Barry prejudice, male prejudice, and class prejudice.

When she died, her death certificate was signed by a man called Staff-Surgeon Major McKinnon, who had never liked her, didn't examine her properly and simply recorded that Dr Barry had died

of diarrhoea. It was not until a charwoman, called Mrs Bishop, laid
out the body that the startling revelation was made. Very startling
it was too, for Mrs Bishop not only said that Dr Barry's body looked
perfectly female, but she maintained that it showed clear signs of
having produced a child — and she knew what she was talking
about she said: she had had nine children herself.

Naturally this story soon found its way into the newspapers, and
it became such a subject of argument that the Registrar General
grew worried about the accuracy of his records and wrote and asked
Dr McKinnon if he had 'ascertained' whether or not Barry was
female. This put McKinnon in an awkward position! But he coun-
tered, most effectively, by using good army tactics and moving into
the attack. Instead of confessing that he had ascertained nothing,
he replied that Barry had died of diarrhoea 'produced apparently
by errors in diet', said that Mrs Bishop was demanding a bribe for
her silence, and — just to make sure everyone overlooked his own
unprofessionalism — gave it as his opinion that Dr Barry had been
a hermaphrodite.[11]

None of this stands up to investigation. Dr Barry did have an
unusual diet, but she had survived on it for a great many years, and
the 'diarrhoea' that had killed her was endemic in London at the
time. Two hundred and sixty-one people died of it during the same
week that she did, and sixteen of them had lived in her neighbourhood. So even McKinnon's statement on the cause of death contains as much prejudice as fact. As for Mrs Bishop (whom McKinnon calls 'the woman'), since she had already had her say and since
her story had become common gossip, she could hardly expect to be
paid for keeping quiet. The hermaphrodite statement is even more
outrageous. What proof did McKinnon have? He hadn't even examined the body. His 'opinion' was clearly a tactical move, based
on his dislike of the eccentric little doctor, and designed to divert
attention from his own incompetence.

Unfortunately, he was successful. The Registrar General accepted
his opinion and so did most of his colleagues. Although a few of
Barry's acquaintances were suddenly finding that they had always
suspected she was a woman, most of them had not suspected anything of the sort, and were not prepared to do so now just because
an ignorant and uneducated charwoman said so. After all, what
right had such a woman to give *any* opinion? She wasn't a doctor.
She was just a working-class nobody.

Besides, Dr Barry *couldn't* have been a woman, for women and medicine were contradictory terms. Although some women had succeeded in graduating in the United States by 1865 — indeed our first truly Canadian medical woman was already in the States studying to become a doctor — all the same, the concept was anathema to the profession. Even if one was forced to admit that it was possible for a woman to get a degree, it was still too much to imagine that any female could perform as brilliantly as Dr Barry had done. So if Barry looked like a woman, there could only be one explanation: she had to be a hermaphrodite.

Today, when we know that women can and do excel in medicine, the whole theory seems ridiculous, especially as Dr Barry had all the characteristics of a very determined female — she was far too extrovert to be convincingly hermaphrodite. But McKinnon's opinion is still given some support, even if it was produced as a cover-up, for Dr Barry did dress as a man and pretend to be one. Why should she do so if she was in fact totally female?

The answer to this question is so obvious that it hardly needs answering. *It was the only way she could become a doctor.*

Edinburgh University would never have accepted a woman. Not in 1809. The very idea would have been considered preposterous. And indeed it was still considered preposterous when, later in the century, women openly began to try to enter university, and — even more ridiculous — said that they wanted to become doctors.

The first Canadians to do so came to a head-on collision with the male establishment. When they knocked hopefully at the doors of Canada's universities, they were told firmly that such institutions of learning were for men only. Girl students would be bad for discipline. Besides, young ladies had no need of higher education. They could learn the piano if they liked and perhaps a little literature and French, but *medicine* — what nonsense! The subject would be way above their heads and, even worse, it would soil their modesty.

So go home, young ladies, and do your duty in that state of life unto which it has pleased God to call you. Our universities have never yet admitted a woman, and they are not going to do so. Ever.

Faced with this attitude, our pioneer women doctors would have found life far easier if they had copied Dr Barry and pretended to be men. But they couldn't do so, partly because many of them tended to plumpness and had large undisguisable bosoms, but mainly because their characters wouldn't permit them to resort to disguise. They wanted to be accepted on their own terms, both in spite of and because they were female. Women, they maintained, were needed as physicians, they had the ability to qualify as physicians, and it was high time this fact was recognized.

So they dressed as women, wearing long Victorian skirts and respectable Victorian hats. And respectable Victorian men took one look at them and went into shock.

2

The suffragist Stowes

IN THESE days of Women's Lib, when we have become acutely sensitive to such issues as The Slights of Women, it is not surprising to find that men were being male chauvinists in the Victorian era. But it is still hard to credit that they could have been so rigidly prejudiced and quite so blatantly unfair — until one realizes that they were fighting desperately for *their* rights.

Women doctors, or prospective doctors as they were at first, were trespassing on male territory, and they represented a most alarming threat. If women were admitted to the professions and — heaven forbid — if they proved equal to the challenge, then the whole law of male supremacy might disintegrate. So the men fought back, and they fought clean or dirty, it didn't matter as long as they won. Some fought by using sarcasm or derision — and women as well as men often joined in the laughter. Others fought by quoting St Paul, or by saying that the Almighty had never intended that women should become physicians. Others fought, most effectively, by simply making it impossible for women to study medicine. And a few — traitors to their sex — thought the whole thing was a most estimable undertaking, and actually aided and abetted these unnatural females.

In spite of the minority support, life was made so difficult for the first medical women that most of them had become rampant suffragettes by the time they had succeeded in graduating. In fact, the first Canadian woman to practise in Canada, Dr Emily Howard Jennings

Stowe, is probably even better known for her suffrage work than she is for being the first Canadian woman doctor. She, more than anyone else, got the women's movement started in Canada. And, although she didn't live to bring in the vote personally, she fought for the cause throughout her life, giving it a powerful injection of Stowe publicity whenever it seemed to be ailing.

One can trace Emily Stowe's feminism directly to the struggle of her early years, but in fact there may always have been a core of suffragette in her, for she was of Quaker stock, and the Quakers not only believed that they should have freedom of worship, they believed in equality for women.[1]

Emily's parents, Hannah Howard Jennings and Solomon Jennings,[2] were American Quakers who had come north to Canada before their marriage, and although their religion developed into Methodism, they retained most of the values of the Society of Friends. So their children would have been brought up with these values. They had six children, all girls, three of whom were to become doctors. (Hannah Augusta Jennings Kimball and Ella Jennings followed the example of their sister Emily and graduated in New York. But they both practised in the States.[3]) Emily, the future Dr Stowe, was the eldest of the family. She was born at Norwich, in Oxford County, Upper Canada in 1831.

Although Norwich was then little more than a pioneering settlement, Emily was given a remarkably thorough education, and she was so effectively encouraged to use it that she started teaching at a small school near Norwich when she was only fifteen.[4] This was a considerable achievement, but it was merely the first step on the road to learning. Soon young Emily Jennings was applying to the University of Toronto — and, of course, being refused. The Senate are said to have 'considered' her application, but the chances are that most of them simply considered it unthinkable.

The Jennings family must have been disappointed, but they can't have been very surprised. Nor were they deterred. This first 'no' from the establishment was treated as a challenge, and in her response to the challenge, Emily was already using the tactics which were to prove so successful in later life. When faced with an obstacle, however insurmountable it seemed, she never retired in dismay. Occasionally she charged in headfirst and battered down the obstacle, but more often she simply went round it, arriving on the other side a little later than should have been necessary — diversions always take more time — but arriving triumphantly nonetheless.

So when Toronto refused her, she determinedly went on teaching until she had saved enough money from her salary to take a year at the Normal School — and when she left the Normal School in 1854, it was with a First Class Teacher's Certificate. This was recognized as so exceptional that she was made principal of Brantford public school — the first woman ever to receive such an appointment in Canada. At the age of twenty-three Emily had already notched up the first of her 'firsts'.

Two years later, in 1856, she married a young Yorkshireman named John Stowe and, at this point, Emily was obliged to pause briefly in her career to give birth to a few children: Ann Augusta Stowe (b. July 1857), John Howard Stowe (b. February 1861) and Frank Jennings Stowe (b. February 1863).[5] The Stowes had moved to Mount Pleasant in Brant County shortly after their marriage and it was there that Emily Stowe taught when she felt able to resume her career. This time she taught in a private school called the Nelles Academy, which — most conveniently — was situated just across the road from her house. Most propitiously too.

The principal of the school was a man called Dr William Waggoner Nelles, and his brother, Dr Samuel Sobiestic Nelles, was the Principal of Victoria College in Cobourg.[6] Significantly, Victoria College was the university which first graduated a woman MD in Canada. And who was this first all-Canadian woman medical graduate? Not Emily Stowe — she had to go to the United States to study — but her daughter Augusta.

One can find most of the why's and wherefore's of Augusta's acceptance by Victoria in the friendship that developed between the Stowe and Nelles families in those early Mount Pleasant days. It was a very active friendship. Emily Stowe taught with Dr William Nelles. John Stowe worshipped with him — John was a Methodist lay preacher and Dr Nelles was a staunch Methodist. John Stowe may even have built Dr Nelles' academy, for he is said to have built his own house, and the two buildings were the only octagonal ones in the neighbourhood. There was certainly a great deal of give and take as the Nelles and Stowe children grew up together, played together, studied together, and as their parents strove together for the enlightenment of the community. So the families were allies as well as friends, and when young Augusta decided that she, too, would become a doctor, obviously the Nelles family did what they could to make her student life easier than her mother's had been.

Emily's student years had been very far from easy. Her return to teaching had been necessity as much as vocation, for her husband developed tuberculosis and had to go into a sanitorium, so she had to support the family. His illness had one merit — it caused Emily to decide to become a doctor — but it also meant that while she was trying to cram for college entrance and save enough money to see her through college, she was also having to work to keep her family in food and clothing — not only for the time being, but for the years she would be away in the States studying medicine. In spite of the friendship with the Nelles family, Victoria College wasn't ready to take women yet. No Canadian college was.

But there was a relatively easy diversion round this obstacle. Dr Elizabeth Blackwell had led the way in the United States by graduating, in 1849, from Geneva Medical College in New York State, and by the second half of the nineteenth century quite a number of American colleges were open to women. So Emily Stowe saved up her salary, left her children in the care of her sister, Cornelia, and set off south to enrol at the New York Medical College for Women,[7] a college which had recently been opened in New York City.

By 1867 Emily Stowe was back in Canada,[8] triumphantly showing off her graduation certificate. This was a magnificent achievement, and she lost no time in putting it to use. She moved her family to Toronto, and soon she was advertising in *The Globe* that Mrs E.H. Stowe, MD, Physician and Accoucheur, would see patients between 9 a.m. and 3 p.m.

Strangely, this wasn't the climax of Emily Stowe's efforts to qualify as a doctor. It was a beginning, the first step in her struggle to be accepted by the profession. Certainly she had won her degree, she had hung up her shingle, set up a practice, and she was gathering a heartening number of patients. But she had not arrived. She wasn't licensed to practise.

In 1869 an Act of Parliament was passed, regularizing the licensing laws and appointing a Council of the College of Physicians and Surgeons of Ontario as the sole licensing board in the province.[9] Dr Stowe applied for registration with the Council — and she was refused. Theoretically, the Council had right on its side: one of its regulations[10] stipulated that graduates from the United States must attend one session of lectures at a recognized Ontario medical school and must also present themselves for a matriculation exam, before the Council would accept their qualifications. Fair enough — except that no Ontario medical school would admit women. So, in effect, this Act debarred women from practising medicine.

It was an absurd situation. Emily Stowe had been forced to graduate in the States because no Canadian university would accept her, and yet by graduating in the States she was still unqualified because no Canadian school of medicine would accept her — not even for one session, which was all that was necessary. There was no way round this obstacle, so Dr Stowe simply ignored it. She had been playing by the rules for long enough. She knew that she was practising illegally, but she also knew that she held an authentic MD certificate, which it had cost her a great deal to achieve, so she saw no reason why she shouldn't call herself a physician and practise as one.

By this time, Dr Stowe's feminism had developed to the stage where she was quite prepared to disobey rules which had been made by males. Crime, she was later to explain, was of two kinds: conventional crime, which merely violated man's laws, and actual crime which transgressed divine law. (By 'man's laws' she meant 'laws and statutes made by man, by male man, as women had had no hand in the compilation of them.'[11])

But if Dr Stowe was prepared to violate the laws laid down by male man, male man wasn't going to sit quietly by and let his laws be violated. One clause in the Ontario Medical Act said that a person could be fined up to a hundred dollars for practising without a licence, or for unlawfully using the name of Physician, Surgeon, Accoucheur, etc. etc. Emily Stowe was almost certainly fined at this time. But there is no record that she stopped practising or that she stopped calling herself a physician. All the same, she did wish to legalize her practice — it would make life so much easier — so she continued to apply for admission to Toronto's medical schools and universities. And her applications continued to be rejected. But she fought back. On one occasion, when she was refused by the University of Toronto, she is said to have replied, most prophetically: 'The day will come when these doors will swing wide open to every female who chooses to apply.'[12]

The doors didn't exactly swing wide open, but Dr Stowe gradu-

ally wore down the opposition and in the early 1870's the doors of
the Toronto School of Medicine were inched open, just a crack, to
allow her and a young woman called Jennie Trout to slip through.
This was a real triumph for Dr Stowe, but it was made to appear as
untriumphant as possible. She was told that she and Mrs Trout
could attend a session of lectures only if they agreed to make no
fuss, *whatever happened*. And of course plenty happened — as the
professors had expected and even hoped.

A friend of Mrs Trout wrote a description of this 'session', and it
sounds horrific enough even now. It must have been an intolerable
experience for those two respectable Victorian ladies:

Little incidents, such as having to observe their seats from a conventional loophole before entering the classroom, lest, as occurred on more
than one occasion, they had to be cleared and cleaned before being
occupied. Other playful activities of some members of the school were
in the way of obnoxious sketches on the wall. There were so many
artists, or at least sketches, that the walls of a classroom had to be
whitewashed four times during that session. But more trying and more
frequent were the needless objectionable stories told by 'enemy' lecturers to the class to instigate its worst element to make noisy and
vulgar demonstration. It was so unbearable on one occasion that one
of the ladies went to the lecturer afterwards and asked him to desist
from that sort of persecution or she would go and tell his wife exactly
what he had said. His lectures were more bearable after that.[13]

After enduring this course of lectures, was Dr Stowe's position
legalized? No, it was not. She was still not given a licence to practise.
The College of Physicians and Surgeons held out against her until
1880.

There are two possible explanations for this action — or lack of
it. One was that Dr Stowe refused to fulfil the second registration
requirement, the examination. It was partly an oral exam, and
it was hardly in Dr Stowe's character to submit to the indignity
of being quizzed by a hostile group of 'male men' — and they
were bound to be hostile. In fact their hostility was so predictable and so uncompromising, that it also explains why Emily's
licence was withheld. This could easily have been as powerful a
factor as her refusal to sit the oral, for she had become public enemy

number one: she had been openly at war with the medical profession for more than a decade, and — even worse — she had won most of the battles.

She had also been extremely active in other even more disreputable schemes. In 1877 she had organized the Toronto Women's Literary Club which was, in effect, a suffragette society.[14] In spite of its harmless name, everyone must have known its purpose. Its meetings were fully reported in the newspapers where, interspersed with accounts of 'instrumental music by Mrs Hamilton' and 'humorous readings by Mrs Wellington', one could read just what Dr E.H. Stowe had to say about the role of women this week. She had a great deal to say. 'Mrs Stowe deprecated the position to which woman has been reduced by the conventionalities of society. . . .' She 'complained that the education of girls just about stops where boys begin to grapple with the abstruser difficulties. . . .'[15]

Mrs Stowe deprecated and complained far too often for the comfort of established society. This stalwart and fearless woman was a dedicated campaigner and her interests had no boundaries. One week she was giving the ladies of her club a lecture on the eye 'illustrated by diagrams and dissection'. Another week she was getting them to write a circular to the Toronto factory owners, 'respectfully drawing their attention to the necessity of supplying separate conveniences (WCs) for each sex.'[16]

The literary society came out into the open in 1883 and called itself the Toronto Women's Suffrage Club. It grew to become the Dominion Women's Enfranchisement Association (1889) and, finally, the Canadian Suffrage Association (1907). By then Emily Stowe had died, but on the great day in 1918 when Canadian women were finally given the federal vote, her name was honoured as one of our greatest suffragettes.

And so she was. However much opposition she may have evoked, however much our fair women and brave men may have disliked this plump and outspoken female with her aggressive lower lip and almost fanatical eyes — which glared out determinedly through round little 'granny glasses' — and however much they may have cringed from That Voice, telling them what they didn't want to know, nevertheless they were all bound to acknowledge in retrospect that she, as much as anyone, had brought about the emancipation of Canadian women. Throughout her life, Dr Stowe never

stopped fighting for the Movement, however occupied she was
with her own affairs, with her family, her practice, or with her
efforts to be recognized as a doctor. And she made sure that everyone in Canada knew that there was a battle being fought.

One of her most publicized efforts towards female suffrage was
the Mock Parliament, which she and her group held in Toronto in
1896.[17] Its purpose was to draw attention to the absurdities of *not*
letting women vote — and it threatened to draw so much attention
that a panic opposition group tried to prevent it taking place. But
as usual, Emily Stowe triumphed, and not only triumphed but
carried off the farce so wittily that even the newspapers decided to
play along with her and report the proceedings good-humouredly.

The suffragettes had hired the Pavilion[18] for their Drama of
Social Import, and there, on February 18 — accompanied by the
Verdi Quartette (Miss Norma Reynolds, Directress) and by refresh-
ments on the European Plan — they let themselves go, pretending
that *they* had always run the country and that it was the men who
were the downtrodden sex. First of all, a deputation of men arrived
(mostly husbands of the 'MPs') and begged that they might be
given the vote. Here was Emily Stowe's chance to get her own back.
She was playing the part of Attorney-General (naturally!) and she
replied to the male deputation with a most convincing imitation
of the real Attorney-General, Sir Oliver Mowat, explaining to
the lowly suppliants that 'although the movement for the enfranchisement of men met with her warmest personal endorsation . . .
even the members of her cabinet, advanced as they were on most
questions, could not see with her in this matter.' However, she
promised to give the matter her serious consideration.

Meanwhile the other ladies were getting their points over too,
bringing out all the well-worn excuses: if we let men into one profession, they'll want to take over the lot; if we let them wear long
stockings when they ride bicycles, they'll want to dress entirely as
women; if we let them into the lighter professions, such as medicine, dressmaking, law and millinery, who will do the physical
labour? We must recognize that, biologically, men are most suited
to the heavy work.

The 'Parliament' was a little forced, but it made its points loud
and clear. And it showed up the absurdities of contemporary reasoning when it transposed the arguments against women to arguments
against men — insisting, for instance, that men had no place in the

professions because they had been designed physically to be hewers of wood and drawers of water. The conventional rationalisations didn't sound quite so rational when they were put this way round.

Emily's husband was a hewer of wood, and he may at times have felt as underprivileged as the male petitioners at the Mock Parliament pretended to be. An 1872 Toronto street directory which lists Emily as Physician, lists John merely as Carriagemaker — definitely a lesser breed. He is a rather shadowy figure, appearing only occasionally behind the dominant Emily, and one cannot tell whether he was proud of his wife's success or slightly jealous of her. But he was probably extremely grateful to her. Emily supported the family while he had tuberculosis, and after his recovery she put him through dental school. By 1878 John was hewing teeth, not wood, and he was appearing in the directories as John Stowe, LDS.[19]

Once John had graduated into the professions, he and Emily ran a joint practice at a house they bought on Church Street. Emily is said to have paid eight thousand dollars[20] for this house, which gives a good indication of her success during the past ten years. Yet in spite of her success, and in spite of the fact that none of her patients had died through malpractice, she had to wait two more years before she received her licence. July 16, 1880, was the day of triumph. It was only then, at the age of forty-nine, that Dr Emily Stowe, MD, Female Physician and Accoucheur, finally won the war she had been fighting for nearly twenty years.

One of the wars. Although women were beginning to be accepted in medicine by this time, there were still other battles to be fought, and after her husband died in 1891 she carried on her campaigns for women's rights with renewed energy. Virtually her entire life was spent fighting for her beliefs.

Few of her beliefs were orthodox. Even her religion experienced a change during her lifetime, partly because the clergy tended to side with the male establishment. Emily Stowe never ceased to be a believer, but she began to call herself a 'scientific socialist' — and that must have alarmed a great many people! She was, she said, a truth seeker, desiring knowledge from the interior life.[21] Even in her death she was different from most people, for she had asked to be cremated (for 'sanitary and convenient motives'). 'I have never done an act on earth to pollute it,' she said to her daughter Augusta, 'and I do not wish to do so in dissolution.'[22]

When Emily died in 1903, the tributes came pouring in, and it is

hard to decide whether she was appreciated mostly for her contribution to the cause of medicine or to the cause of women. 'Your
mother was a pioneer in every sense of the word,' Susan B. Anthony,
who had recently resigned as president of the National American
Woman Suffrage Association, wrote to Augusta. Emily would have
agreed with this. In 1896 she had written: 'My career has been
one of much *struggle* characterized by the usual persecution which
attends every*one* who pioneers a new movement or steps out of line
with established custom.'[23]

She had indeed pioneered a new movement. Several. And fortunately she had also bred a daughter who was eager to carry on
where she left off.

Even in the early days of the Women's Literary Club, young
Augusta Stowe was making her presence felt and her voice heard:

Miss Stowe claimed for her sex equal rights with men in the matter of
work and wages. . . . She also claimed that women were as wise and
judicious rulers as men, were not as selfish or ambitious, and gave a
lengthy list of notable women from the time of Cleopatra and Zenobia
to Queen Victoria.[24]

After a promising beginning, Augusta Stowe became increasingly
more active in the suffrage movement: in the Mock Parliament she
sat on the front bench as a cabinet minister. And, like her mother,
she also decided to become a doctor.

Qualifying as a doctor wasn't easy for Augusta, but it was considerably easier than it had been for her mother. In 1879, when
Augusta sat the matriculation exam of the College of Physicians and
Surgeons (a prerequisite for anyone who wanted to study medicine), the idea of accepting women at universities wasn't as shocking as it used to be. Queen's College at Kingston was planning to
start a course especially for women, and at Victoria College in
Cobourg, Principal Nelles was looking with a kindly eye on the
ambitions of his young friend, Augusta Stowe.

Having passed her matriculation, Augusta chose Victoria College.
This may have been for family reasons, but it may also have been
for professional reasons. By enrolling at Victoria, Augusta would
be part of the mainstream instead of in a possible backwater — for
the Queen's course was a summer affair for women only. Besides, en-

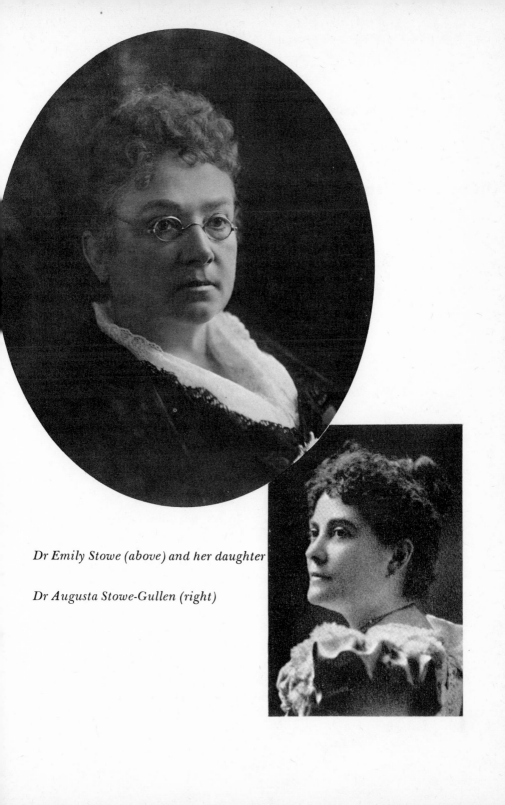

Dr Emily Stowe (above) and her daughter

Dr Augusta Stowe-Gullen (right)

rolment at Cobourg meant, surprisingly, that Augusta could live at home: at that time Victoria medical students took their classes at the Toronto School of Medicine.

Whatever the reasons for Augusta's choice of university, it was a most fortunate decision, for it made her the first Canadian woman to get a medical degree in Canada. Although three young women were studying medicine at Kingston while Augusta was studying medicine in Toronto, their classes were shifted around so much with curriculum alterations and a change to winter instead of summer sessions that they lost a year and didn't graduate until 1884. Meanwhile Augusta had proudly graduated as Canada's First in 1883.

In spite of this great honour, which she was so justly proud of in later years, Augusta must often have wished that she had joined the Queen's girls or, at least, that she had female company in her classes. It wasn't pleasant to be the only girl among a gang of young medical students. A speech made on Augusta's graduation compliments her by saying that 'although she had received her instruction in a mixed class of both sexes, there had never existed the slightest difficulty in the class owing to her presence there.'[25] But there were difficulties, as the same speech admits when it tells how the whole class championed her cause when 'an attempt had been made to create some disturbance.'

She didn't have to submit to such a campaign of hate as her mother and Mrs Trout had done, but the same tactics were used by both students and lecturers. By some of them at any rate. According to Augusta's family, she often cried all the way home from college, and then cried herself to sleep at night. But she was a true Stowe and when the going got really tough, she launched into the attack and told one particularly offensive student exactly what she thought of him. After this the boys treated her more warily, and by the time she graduated she was one of the most popular members of the class. In fact she had become so popular with one of her classmates — John Benjamin Gullen — that he had asked her to marry him.

The Stowe-Gullen wedding took place within a week of the graduation ceremony, the invitations proudly announcing that Dr Augusta Stowe was going to marry Dr John B. Gullen. According to the newspapers, it was a splendid affair, 'largely attended by the

intellectual elite of Toronto and by the bride's aunt, Mrs Judge
Tilden of Cleveland, O.' Mrs Judge Tilden was Emily's sister Cornelia, who had looked after the Stowe children for so many years,
and, in spite of the newspaper report, she may have been just as
elitist intellectually as the Toronto guests: in her later years she
became a collector for an American gallery,[26] going on trips to
Europe to see what she could find — dressed incongruously in traditional Quaker clothing. No member of that family could possibly
be *ordinary*. And, of course, the doctors Gullen didn't have an
ordinary honeymoon. They went straight off to New York to take
a postgraduate course in children's diseases.

When they returned from New York, Augusta Stowe-Gullen was
appointed Demonstrator of Anatomy at the Woman's Medical College which had recently been established in Toronto, largely at her
mother's instigation. It must have been a very exciting time for her
— to graduate and marry and be given a teaching position, all in one
year. It would be a heady enough achievement nowadays, but in
1883 it was an unprecedented one, and young Augusta was well
aware of this as she conscientiously took up her duties at the medical
college.

The Woman's Medical College was just starting its life in 1883
and it represented a real breakthrough, as did the Kingston Women's Medical College which was founded at the same time. All
along, developments in Kingston had paralleled those in Toronto,
sometimes moving a little ahead, sometimes behind, marching in
rivalry rather than in step. So when the breakthrough came, it
came with double impact and prospective women doctors found
that they actually had a choice of college. Since there was only a
handful of students at either college to begin with, two separate
establishments were not by any means necessary, but that was beside
the point. The point was that at last girls could study to become
doctors without being persecuted. And they could do so in an all-
female environment.

The two women's medical colleges were welcomed by the public
and given good support, for attitudes had been changing during the
past few years. The idea of women in medicine was no longer so
alarming. In fact, in those days of extreme modesty, many women
were only too pleased to be able to consult a lady doctor. Yet it was
this obsession with modesty that had proved the chief barrier against

women *becoming* doctors, for the classes had necessarily been co-educational and that hadn't been considered at all tasteful. Although the more progressive academics (and the pioneer women had always received *some* support) had felt that the end justified the means, most people had only been able to see the means. Or rather, they only saw some of the means. What they mostly seem to have seen, or imagined, was pretty young girls and handsome young men working together to dissect the sexual organs of some cadaver. Disgusting!

We should be sorry indeed [wrote a Kingston paper] to know that Canadian maidens, or matrons either, were so dead to that modesty which is woman's chief charm, as to sit unmoved side by side with young men, and listen to lectures on obstetrics or anatomy, witnessing the experiments of one or the experiments in the other. . . . To think of disclosing the human form divine, over which humanity bids us throw a veil of decency, or of having the most sacred of feminine mysteries freely discussed before a mixed class of young men and young women is not only shocking, but is disgusting and degrading.[27]

The editors of the Kingston paper obviously didn't agree with the article, since they subtitled it 'A Strange Opinion', but there is no doubt that it represented a prevalent attitude. After all, Victorians were obsessed with the purity of womanhood. Young ladies were expected to be refined and delicate — and shielded from anything that was gross or offensive. Considering the extremely offensive experience of childbirth at the time, this attitude now seems ridiculously hypocritical, but it was a hypocritical age. It was an age when some families even clothed their table legs in frills, because naked legs of any type were considered 'disgusting and degrading'. And it was a repressed age — which explains why the young medical students behaved so badly when they found they had women in their class. These women had broken the modesty barrier, so, with relief, the young men let themselves go and shattered it into fragments. They almost shattered the women too.

It was predictable that the two women who had sat through the first co-educational course — Dr Stowe and Dr Trout — should be the founding spirits behind the two medical colleges. They had suffered and they had survived, but it was time to put a stop to this nonsense. So they went about their plans, jointly at first, and then separately — Emily Stowe in Toronto and Jennie Trout in Kingston.

In Toronto, Dr Stowe had a good deal of support, especially from Dr Michael Barrett, the Professor of Physiology at Toronto, who was as eager to get a women's college started as she was. He had been one of the 'friendly' lecturers at the Toronto School of Medicine — no offences had been committed in his classes—but of course he had heard of the student outrages. So he too felt that such nonsense should stop and that a women's medical college should be established, and it was he who formally outlined the proposal at a meeting of Emily Stowe's suffrage group in June, 1883.[28]

This meeting is interesting, since it shows that at last Emily Stowe was joining forces with the male establishment. There was an impressive array of speakers present. Mr. Justice Patterson was in the Chair, and the meeting was attended by such upright figures as Mr James Beatty, QC, MP, the Rev John King, DD, Dr James Carlyle, Professor Thomas Kirkland — and, of course, by Dr Michael Barrett, MA, MD, who was to be the Dean of the new college. The college certainly had solid backing, and after some initial difficulties, it got off to a promising start when it was inaugurated, in October, by His Worship the Mayor of Toronto, Mr A.R. Boswell.

From then on it never looked back, though it had financial worries from time to time. During its twenty-three years of life, the college qualified more than one hundred doctors, and when it closed its doors in 1906, it only did so because the University of Toronto had agreed to accept women. Attitudes had become more 'liberal' and a separate women's college was no longer felt to be necessary.

But women's colleges were essential in the 1880's and it was most fitting that this particular college should appoint Dr Augusta Stowe-Gullen as its first female staff member: her mother had helped found it, and besides, young Dr Stowe-Gullen was the only woman who had graduated in medicine in Canada. At first she was the only female staff member at the college, but her appointment was more than tokenism. It was part of the feminist policy of the college to include women in the administration, and by 1906, women represented one third of the staff. But Augusta remained the leader, the most powerful female voice, and she steadily rose to become Professor of Diseases of Children, President of the Alumnae Association, and one of the directors of the College.

Like her mother, Augusta had tremendous energy. And like her mother, she didn't confine her interests to one field. While she was teaching at the medical college, she ran a practice at her home on Spadina Road and — as if this wasn't enough to fill her time — she also worked at the Western Hospital. Her husband, John, was one of the founders of the Western, so Augusta was actively involved in it from the beginning, and even delivered its first baby.

This baby was born on November 1, 1896 — rather prematurely for the hospital, which was little more than a dispensary at the time, and had neither the furniture nor the equipment suitable for a natal clinic. But this didn't deter young Mrs Dr Stowe-Gullen. The baby was delivered successfully and, having dealt with *that* emergency, she moved on busily to see what else needed doing, and was soon forming a ladies' committee, made up of the wives of doctors, to provide the hospital with linens and equipment. This committee was known as the Women's Board and it became a type of corporate godmother to the nurses: one of its achievements was to provide the nurses with their present residence. Augusta served as its president until 1928 when she retired from it in graceful glory, with many appreciative speeches and with a magnificent silver tea service in acknowledgement of her painstaking work.[29]

That was just one of the committees Augusta worked on. She was a very energetic committee woman and there seems to have been little that she didn't belong to. From 1892 to 1896 she served on the Toronto School Board, she was Vice-President of the Ontario Social Service Council, Honorary President of the Canadian Suffrage Association, a member of the University Women's Club, of the Women's Art Association . . . and she was also appointed to represent the medical profession on the Senate of the University of Toronto. To top it all off, she was awarded the King's Medal in 1935.[30]

This impressive list of honours makes it very clear that Augusta Stowe-Gullen lived far more within society than her mother had ever done. By the end of Emily Stowe's life, she might have been considered one of Society's pillars. But Augusta was always more than a pillar: she was a cornerstone. She became one of Toronto's

most respected public figures — to such an extent that she could
hardly utter an opinion on *anything* without it being reported by
the Press.

Many of her opinions were surprisingly conventional. When
asked what she thought of the short skirts and silk stockings worn
by the flapper generation, she condemned them strongly. She based
her disapproval on medical reasons: she had had to treat several
young girls for frozen limbs during the winter. Short skirts
didn't give enough protection, she said.[31] They showed a lack of
common sense among the young. Fair enough. Yet she was prepared
to dress in the equally senseless fashions of a former age. Most of
her portraits show her in full-length, ornate dresses, which have
been pulled in at the waist to the point of discomfort. She loved
attractive clothes and would sacrifice quite a bit of comfort, and
cash, in order to appear at dinners in suitable splendour.

Having heard Dr Stowe-Gullen's opinion on short skirts, it is no
surprise to find her nephew writing that she was a 'stickler for eti-
quette'.[32] Yet one simply cannot class Augusta Stowe-Gullen
among those who won't move with the times. She and her husband
were among the first Toronto people to have a car (a Babcock
Electric, licence number 6). She was well up to date there. And in
many respects she was way ahead of her times. She was advocating
that women should receive half their husband's salary in the days
when a woman's entire fortune was considered the property of her
husband. And though she was so conventional in her clothing, she
was prepared to dress up in bloomers, jacket and cap, and ride a
bicycle down Yonge Street — just to show that women had the same
rights as men.

There were similar contradictions in her religion. She was proud
of her Quaker ancestry and yet she hated St Paul — 'that man' who
said that women should subject themselves unto their husbands.
And although she had been brought up as a Methodist, she had
foresworn all religions by the end of her life and was far more interested in Spiritualism[33] than in The Holy Spirit — she used to
have a great time table-turning at the Stowe property in Muskoka.
It was one of her few relaxations.

Both Augusta and John Gullen lived into their eighties, which
meant that they were able to celebrate the diamond jubilee of both
their wedding and their graduation. It was a fitting climax to a life-

time of medical work. Together with her husband, Augusta Stowe-Gullen had made an impressive and indelible mark on Canadian medicine. As a Gullen, she had helped establish the Western Hospital. As a Stowe, she had not only helped establish women in medicine, but she personally had blazed the trail.

The Stowe family did so much for medical women and *as* medical women that they have come to be accepted as The Pioneers. But they were not the only women in the field, nor were they the only firsts. While Augusta was studying at the Toronto School of Medicine, three of her contemporaries were studying at Queen's. And when Dr Stowe was getting her college started in Toronto, Dr Trout was establishing a similar college at Kingston.

The three Queen's students are well known and have been given almost as much publicity as Augusta, but Dr Trout is a more puzzling character. She is mentioned from time to time, but never with any consistency. In fact, she is so often not mentioned that one begins to feel that there was some mystery about her. This air of mystery thickens into a fog when one begins to look through Emily Stowe's scrapbook of newspaper clippings. One of the cuttings mentions Jennie Trout — and her name has been crossed out heavily, almost angrily, in thick blue ink. What could Dr Trout have done to warrant such complete obliteration?

SEVEN GRADUATES OF THE TORONTO
WOMAN'S MEDICAL COLLEGE

ANNIE ELLA CARVETH HIGBEE
(MD CM Trinity, 1893)

Annie Carveth (Mrs Higbee) has gained renown for many achievements — not
the least being that she lived to be 100 years old.

She was born in Port Hope in 1864, and after graduating she practised in
Windsor for a short time before moving to California — for health reasons —
and meeting and marrying Charles E. Higbee, a high school principal.
Dr Higbee practised in California until 1912 when, with her husband and her
son John, she moved north — quite far north — to a 640 acre farm some way
out of Grande Prairie in the Peace River District of Alberta. There, 'Dr Annie'
took up the role of horse-and-buggy homesteading doctor, sometimes travelling
as much as 20 miles in one night to deliver a baby. In summer she travelled
by horse, her instruments strapped to the saddle, and in winter she travelled
in a one-horse sleigh, driven by her son. In this manner she regularly covered
long distances as she visited her scattered patients or visited her office — which
was in Grande Prairie, fifteen miles from the Higbee homestead.

Dr Higbee's third career began in 1919 when the family moved to Toronto.
Her brother, Dr George Carveth, had been one of the founders of the Western
Hospital and Annie joined the staff as an anaesthetist. She retired from the
Western in 1929 at the age of 65 — but she was not yet ready to retire from
medicine. She practised in Newcastle until 1939.

EMILY JANET IRVINE SMITH
(MB Toronto, 1890).

Emily Irvine (Mrs Smith) was of United Empire Loyalist Stock. She was born
in Woodstock and practised medicine for some years in Brampton and
Toronto.

EVA JEANETTE RYAN FISHER
(MD CM Trinity, 1893)

Eva Ryan (Mrs Fisher) was one of the many women who taught school in
order to raise the fees for their medical studies. After graduation, she practised
in Arthur for 35 years, and she was in charge of the Red Cross Hospital in
Tobermory for 4 years.

ANNIE MACKENZIE CHAMBERS CLELAND
(MD CM Trinity, 1892)
Annie Chambers (Mrs Cleland) practised in Victoria and was one of the first
women to be licensed in British Columbia.

HARRIETTA (Etta) PATERSON DENOVAN
(MD CM Victoria, 1892)
Etta Paterson (Mrs Denovan) was one of the medical pioneers in Alberta,
when it was still part of the North-West Territories. She and her husband, the
Rev Dr H.J. Denovan, practised at Red Deer from 1895 to 1903.

NANCY RODGER CHENOWETH
(MD CM Trinity, 1894)
Nancy Rodger (Mrs Chenoweth) was a pioneer both in Alberta (then part
of the North-West Territories) and in British Columbia. Like Dr Denovan,
she was married to a minister, and she practised as part of her husband's
Methodist ministry, first at Walsh, near Medicine Hat, then at Pincher Creek
and finally at Michel, B.C. After her husband died, in 1911, she took a course
in X-ray at the University of Chicago, and practised in Michigan where she
became famed for her X-ray work: patients were sent to her from 200 miles
away in order to be given a special investigation with her 'machine'.

MARGARET BLAIR GORDON
(MD CM Trinity, 1898)
Dr Gordon became one of the most famous women doctors of her time, being
especially well known for her suffrage work. For about ten years she was
Vice-President of the Canadian Suffrage Association, and for a while she was
also President of the Toronto Suffrage Association. She died in 1928.

3

Jennie Trout moves ahead

ALTHOUGH Jennie Kidd Trout was one of our earliest women doctors, today she is seldom given much attention, or even recognized as a pioneer. History has taken its tone from the Stowe family and virtually crossed her off the record, mentioning her only occasionally and then in a random manner, or writing of her anonymously as 'another lady' who attended lectures with Emily Stowe. Dr Trout isn't even considered important enough to be mentioned in the encyclopaedias. Look up *Stowe* in one of them, and you may find several paragraphs about Dr Emily, but look up *Trout* in the same encyclopaedia, and what do you find? A long article about fish. But it isn't really surprising that Jennie Trout is so little known today. When she died in 1921, the *Canadian Medical Association Journal* didn't even record the fact. Already she had been forgotten.

Since Dr Trout was so quickly forgotten, and so thoroughly, it would be natural to assume that she was not a very notable character, that Emily Stowe was the great pioneer — as indeed she was — and that Dr Trout just happened to be around too. But the contemporary records contradict this impression. During the years when Jennie Trout was practising in Toronto, her name is mentioned far too often — and with too much respect — for her to be discounted simply as an 'also ran'. Here she is in *The Globe* managing something called the Electro-Therapeutic Institute. Here she is in the Calendar of the Kingston Women's Medical College — 'Our Benefactor' and 'Our Distinguished Friend'. Here she is in an 1877 book on the Notabilities of Toronto. And here she is in the 1878 Ontario Medical Register: Jennie K. Trout, registered with the College of Physicians and Surgeons of Ontario, May 13, 1875 (the same year that she graduated from the Woman's Medical College of Pennsylvania).

It doesn't take any great feat of mental arithmetic to work out that 1875 was five years *before* 1880 when Dr Stowe was registered. Jennie Trout must therefore have been the first woman licensed to practise medicine in Canada.

Our first licensed woman doctor, yet hardly any biographies mention her? It doesn't make sense — unless she was American. But she wasn't. She was as Canadian as Sir John A. Macdonald. Like him, like so many of our pioneers, she had been born in Scotland and brought to Canada as a small child.[1] But, unlike Sir John A. Macdonald, Dr Trout had no ambition to become a national figure, or even a public figure — and here is the explanation of how she was so easily overlooked. She disliked publicity. It is as simple as that. And she disliked publicity to such an extent that she consciously avoided the role of celebrity.

'She never had any interest in Society,' her brother-in-law wrote of her, she 'was always disposed to retirement and seclusion.'[2] Considering the unsecluded nature of much of Dr Trout's life, this seems a very strange epitaph, but it does explain how she faded so quickly from the limelight after her retirement. Although she would advertise herself during her active years and even seek out publicity in order to achieve what she believed she had been put on earth to achieve, she didn't really enjoy being a public figure. Fame was not an end, it was a means, and when it could no longer serve a purpose, it ceased to be important.

But in spite of her retiring nature, Dr Trout was very well known at one time, and she might still be well known today if there hadn't been another force at work: the rival opposition. Although Dr Stowe died long before Dr Trout did, Emily Stowe had a daughter who remained very much alive, who outlived Jennie Trout by more than twenty years, who became a prominent member of Toronto's professional and social circles, who lectured, made speeches, wrote pamphlets — and who told the story of the early medical women almost exclusively as a Stowe story, mentioning Dr Trout only when it was unavoidable, and then merely as an adjunct to Dr Emily.

All this clearly explains how Dr Trout came to be overshadowed by Dr Stowe, but it doesn't entirely explain why. For instance, it doesn't explain why Augusta so seldom mentioned her mother's friend. One could put it down to Augusta's family pride — a natural desire to represent her mother as the only memorable pioneer — but that page in the Stowe scrapbooks suggests that there was more to it than this: it suggests that the omission of Dr Trout's name was intentional. And that there was quite a bit of feeling behind it too.

Most of the newspaper clippings in the scrapbook have been glued firmly into the book, mistakes and all, without even a pencil correction, yet this particular clipping[3] has been edited in thick blue ink. The offending sentence reads: 'Dr Emily Stowe (with her friend Mrs Trout) had, sometime in the seventies, forced her way to a season's lectures on chemistry' — and the entire bracketed phrase has been crossed out. But Jennie Trout did attend a season's lectures in the seventies. And she did so with Dr Stowe. The lectures weren't specifically on chemistry — it was a medical course that the two women attended — but if the editor had been correcting for accuracy, why didn't she simply delete the word 'chemistry'? And why was the word 'friend' crossed out too? As part of the parenthesis? Or because Dr Trout was no longer considered a friend?

It is an intriguing clue, or non-clue, because there is plenty of evidence to show that the Doctors Stowe and Trout were very close friends at one time. Jennie Trout was only ten years younger than Emily Stowe — she was born in 1841[4] — and she saw a great deal of Emily when she was first in Toronto. The Trout family business and the Stowe house were in the same block on Church Street,[5] only a few steps from each other, and Toronto was so small in those days that the two women couldn't have avoided being on visiting terms. But in any case they had so much in common that they would naturally have been drawn together. Both were intelligent, dedicated women who were striving for the same cause. Both had taught school as young women. Both were energetic and vocal feminists. And both had chosen medicine as a career.

Their backgrounds had been similar too. Although Jennie had been born at Kelso in Scotland, she was only six years old when her parents, Andrew and Elizabeth Gowanlock, emigrated to Canada. They had settled a few miles north of Stratford — not so very far from where Emily's parents had settled — and Jennie passed her childhood in a small rural community, much as Emily had done. In Stratford, as in Norwich, the pioneering spirit was strong. In these small settlements in Upper Canada, success only came with effort, and children were brought up to make that effort. The Gowanlock's farm was some way out of Stratford,[6] where Jennie went to school, and in those days there was no school bus to whisk children to their lessons. The young girl had to make her own way to school, through mud, dust or snow, depending on the season. Yet Jennie attended regularly and did her lessons eagerly, just as Emily had done a decade earlier.

It is interesting that the pattern of Jennie Gowanlock's life during this period repeats Emily Jennings' almost point by point. Like Emily, young Jennie did well at school. Like Emily, she passed into the Normal School. Like Emily, she passed out of it with a teacher's certificate. And then she taught school in Stratford until, in 1865, she married.[7]

But here the pattern begins to change. Jennie Gowanlock married a young man called Edward Trout, an ambitious young man who intended to make his way in the world. Edward[8] had earned his first money by giving writing classes in various Ontario towns, which was probably how he first met Jennie with the light brown hair, but he wasn't content to remain a teacher. Within a few years, he was working for the Leader Printing Company as well as running a commercial college in Toronto. This was the beginning of a most successful career, which curved sharply upwards when Edward joined his brother, John, to found and publish the *Monetary Times*. At first, Edward ran the business side of the journal — bookkeeping was his real talent — but when his brother died in 1876, Edward took over as editor. And from then on his fortunes flourished.

But his wife did not flourish. Not at first. Periodically, during her life, Jennie suffered from 'nervous bodily ailments' and the first six years of her marriage were spent between bed and sofa, struggling to feel well enough to *do* something with her education. She might have remained an invalid for life if a friend of hers, Amelia

Tefft,[9] hadn't persuaded her to try electrotherapeutics, a treatment
which was highly considered at the time and which proved so effec-
tive that Jennie became well enough to live a normal life again. In
fact she became well enough to live an abnormal life, for during
those years of sickness, she had realized that she wanted to take up
medicine.

Amelia Tefft had constantly encouraged Mrs Trout to do so —
and there was somebody else who had been encouraging her too:
Emily Stowe. Indeed, Emily Stowe may have given Jennie Trout
more than encouragement, for in the early 1870's when Edward
Trout was still establishing himself in Toronto, the Trouts had
moved into 135 Church Street — and the Stowes had been living at
135 Church Street since 1869. So there may, from the start, have
been a debt of gratitude in the relationship between the women.
But in those early days, when the Trouts were living with the
Stowes, it doesn't seem to have complicated the friendship. The
two women were staunch companions. Together they discussed
women's rights. Together they braved the Toronto School of Medicine. And together they discussed Jennie's future as a doctor. It was
while she was living at Church Street that Jennie Trout had her
first medical education, and it was from Church Street that she set
off for Philadelphia in 1872[10] to study at the Woman's Medical
College of Pennsylvania. All with Emily Stowe's approval and
support.

But in 1875, when Jennie Trout returned from Philadelphia as
a Doctor of Medicine, she moved out from under the Stowe um-
brella, for she could stand on her own now, and set up her own
practice. In preparation for doing so, she applied for registration
with the College of Physicians and Surgeons.

According to that Act — the licensing Act that had proved such a
barrier to Dr Stowe — Jennie Trout would have to take a course at
an Ontario medical school and the matriculation exam of the
Council of the College of Physicians and Surgeons, before she could
be registered in Ontario. She had already sat through the medical course, in her fiery ordeal with Dr Stowe at the Toronto School
of Medicine, so all that stood between her and her licence was a
simple exam. Or a fearsome exam. But in fact it proved to be
very unfearsome. The College of Physicians and Surgeons seems
to have treated the young woman most gallantly, and when Edward

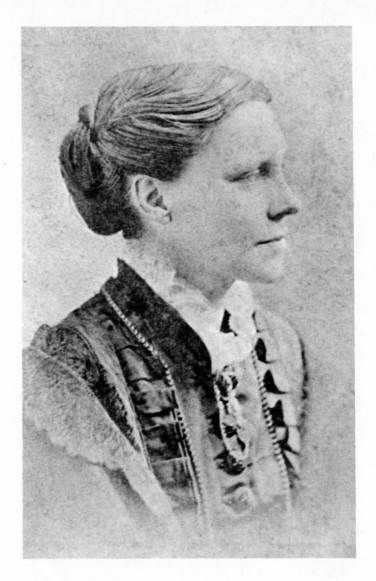

Dr Jennie Trout

Trout called to collect Jennie after her oral, he was complimented
on having such a talented wife who had passed her exams so
creditably.[11]

Whether or not Emily Stowe complimented Dr Trout so warmly
is not known. She had still not submitted to the exam, and she was
still not licensed. But then she was not as submissive a character as
Dr Trout. Nor was she so pragmatic. Although Jennie Trout was
just as dedicated a feminist as Emily Stowe ever was, she didn't let
her enthusiasm for the Cause outweigh her common sense — and
she realized that the registration laws had not been passed especially
to keep women out of medicine. They had been passed to make
quite sure that people who called themselves Doctor would be
worthy of the title. Male as well as female graduates from the States
were required to sit one session at an Ontario medical school *and*
the exam if they wished to be licensed to practise in Ontario. So
Jennie Trout was willing to sit the exam. And delighted to receive
her licence.

By rights, Emily Stowe should have been suffering a serious
attack of schizophrenia when this happened, half of her applauding
her friend's success, and the other half hating it. For years she had
been fighting for the acceptance of women in medicine, and Jennie
Trout had been accepted. Very good. For years she had been encouraging Jennie Trout to become a doctor, and now Jennie Trout
was a doctor. Also very good. But Emily Stowe liked to be the
leader, and Jennie Trout was no longer following her lead. The
younger woman had made her own decision to fulfil the registration
requirements, and she was now setting up her own practice in a
manner that looked as if it might overshadow Dr Stowe's. The
protegée was fast becoming a prodigy.

For some time, Emily had been advertising in *The Globe* each
Tuesday, Thursday and Saturday:

> Emily H. STOWE, MD, FEMALE PHYSICIAN
> No. 135 Church st, Toronto
> Office hours 12 to 4 p.m.

Then, one morning in 1875, a rival announcement appeared under
her own:

MRS TROUT, GRADUATE OF
the Woman's Medical College of Pennsylvania,
member of the College of Physicians and Surgeons,
Ont., Office 272 Jarvis-st. Special facilities
for giving treatment to ladies by galvanic
baths or electricity. Office hours 11 to 12 a.m.
and 2 to 4 p.m.[12]

Emily wouldn't have been human if she hadn't felt some small twinge of envy. She too began to offer her patients electrical treatment, but she didn't go in for it on such a large scale.

Jennie Trout had been interested in electrical treatment ever since her friend, Amelia Tefft, had encouraged her to try it for her own illness, and by 1877 she was running an establishment called the Therapeutic and Electrical Institute (proprietors Trout and Tefft), with Amelia Tefft as the junior partner.[13] Miss Tefft was an old friend and companion of the Trouts, and she had accompanied Jennie to Philadelphia, studied with her, and also graduated MD, so here was another pioneer in the field. But there is no record that Dr Tefft was ever licensed to practise in Ontario. As the junior partner in the Institute, she may not have needed a licence, but in any case it was possible to practise without one, even if it wasn't legal. Dr Stowe had proved that clearly enough — and she had a thriving practice.

Nevertheless, Dr Stowe wasn't functioning in such a grand manner as Dr Trout. Edward Trout had been doing well in the past few years. As a partner in the firm Odell and Trout, as partner in the firm J.M. Trout & Co., and as Editor of the *Monetary Times and Trade Review*, he was in a position to set his wife up in style. The Therapeutic and Electrical Institute occupied four lots on Jarvis Street — 272 to 278 — and it housed about sixty patients. The rooms were well heated and contained a great many baths and expensive electrical apparatus, and the whole place seems to have been lavishly decorated. A young friend of Dr Trout continually used such words as 'magnificent' and 'ample' when describing the Jarvis Street Institute.[14] On one visit, she was conducted through 'splendidly furnished parlors . . . up stairs through brilliantly furnished apartments to an exquisite bedroom' to lay aside her wraps — and she noted that even the food was delicious and of more than ample supply.

Yet in spite of all this magnificence, the young visitor was mostly impressed by Dr Trout herself, remembering her gentleness and her large kindly eyes. Jennie Trout was extremely religious and, at the height of her success, she remained a gentle, sweet-natured woman whose main concern was helping others. And it wasn't only her patients that she was helping in the splendid Jarvis Street building. She had taken in several young girls — friends or relatives — and was giving them a home, encouragement, training, or whatever they most needed.

The Electro-Therapeutic Institute continued until 1882, when it closed down, partly because it wasn't a financial success[15] — Edward had done a bit of bookkeeping. But the main reason for its closure was that the pressure of work was proving too much of a strain on Jennie Trout's health. Her registration with the College in 1875 had been so widely publicized that she must have been appalled (even though she had encouraged the publicity by advertising in *The Globe*); she had suddenly sprung to fame, and had been deluged with letters from women asking for treatment. She had responded all too vigorously. During the past few years, besides managing her Institute, she had been running a free dispensary for the poor where she saw at least fourteen patients a day, she had established branch offices in Hamilton and Brantford, and she had been travelling round Ontario giving lectures on medicine.[16] All this in addition to anything she might be doing for non-medical causes. For a period she was Vice-President of the Association for the Advancement of Women, and she was also President of the Woman's Temperance Union. Quite a handful for a woman who, by nature, liked 'retirement and seclusion'!

Even after the Jarvis Street institute closed, Dr Trout didn't retire from the scene completely for there was still necessary work to be done. In 1882 neither of the women's medical colleges had yet been established, and this became Dr Trout's next objective: to organize and endow a college for the medical education of women.

At first she set her sights on Toronto, working with the Stowes and offering to give ten thousand dollars towards setting up a women's college in the city.[17] But she met obstacles. Or, rather, she presented them, for she was only prepared to give the ten thousand if women sat on the governing board of the college and if women were admitted to the staff. She felt it was only fitting that women should play an active role in running a women's medical college.

The academics of Toronto didn't agree with her. Even Emily Stowe's friend, Dr Barrett, wouldn't go along with the suggestion. So . . . rather than compromise and get a women's college started at any cost, Jennie Trout transferred her attention to Kingston where there was an equally reputable university and medical school which might sponsor a women's college.

Queen's was more receptive to the idea of professional women than the Toronto universities had been, for they desperately needed a women's college. Ever since the Queen's summer course had been started in 1880, Queen's had been committed to educating a few women in medicine — yet this wasn't proving at all easy. In fact it was proving extremely difficult, for the university had recently been shaken by an alarming outbreak of student unrest, which threatened to destroy the medical school unless the women students were dismissed. So neither town nor gown were in any mood to quibble over details. Dr Trout's proposal was welcomed with relief and a meeting was called at Kingston's City Council Chamber on June 8, 1883. Proposals were made, donations received, and plans were drawn up to open a women's medical college in the fall.

This meeting was well reported in the newspapers, so there was no excuse for the meeting which took place in Toronto a few days later.

On June 11, only three days after the Kingston meeting, the academics of Toronto decided that they would agree to have women on the staff after all, and on June 13 they held *their* meeting — the meeting that was organized by Dr Stowe's suffrage group — to set up a women's medical college in Toronto. Along with the impressive list of doctors, reverends, lawyers and judges who attended Dr Stowe's meeting, Edward Trout, publisher, was also present, loudly defending his wife and accusing the Torontonians of being copycats. He said that 'the calling of a meeting at this late date was an act of discourtesy toward the Kingston people.'[18] The Kingston group, he said, had waited patiently until they saw that there was no chance of a Toronto school succeeding. They had then gone ahead, formed committees, received subscriptions, got the whole thing rolling to set up a women's college on a 'liberal basis' . . . and now, only a few days after it had all been signed and sealed, Toronto had decided to plan a liberal-based women's college too. It was both insulting and unnecessary.

And so it was. There weren't enough prospective women medical students to warrant the expense of setting up two separate colleges in the same province. There was no need for the Toronto college.

No need, but plenty of reasons. Could Toronto allow itself to revert to 'muddy York' and take second place to Kingston? Could the University of Toronto let Queen's take the lead? And — equally significant — could Emily Stowe let Jennie Trout take the lead?

Since her graduation, Jennie Trout had been gaining ground steadily over Emily Stowe. As pioneer, patron and practitioner, *she* was becoming the grand old lady of medicine. How thoroughly this was happening can be gauged from looking at Henry Morgan's *The Canadian Men and Women of the Time.* In the first edition, Dr Stowe is featured as the woman pioneer, and there is no mention of Dr Trout. But Dr Stowe has been dropped from the second edition and she has been replaced by Dr Trout who, says Morgan, 'enjoys the honour of being the first woman who qualified to practice med. in Can.'[19]

True enough, because Emily Stowe wasn't qualified until she was registered, but it is doubtful if the Stowes found the statement true. Or just. After all, Emily Stowe had been practising for thirteen years before she was registered. She was practising when Jennie Trout was only *thinking* of becoming a doctor. So what right had Jennie Trout to come along and usurp the position of pioneer, just because male man had decided to add a few letters after her name? Talk about ingratitude! Why, if it hadn't been for Emily, Jennie might never have become a doctor.

Looked at in this light, it is not surprising that Augusta Stowe-Gullen didn't go out of her way to praise Dr Trout's work when she gave lectures on the early days of medicine. And it is not surprising that Emily Stowe had to sponsor her own medical college either. As it turned out, the Toronto college was inaugurated one day before the Kingtson one (it opened on October 1, while the Kingston women's college opened on October 2) but historians have chosen to ignore this piece of one-upmanship. Both colleges are recorded as having started at the same time: October, 1883.

Since both colleges were set up on a 'liberal basis', both included women among their governors. And the staff was to include women too. In Toronto, Augusta Stowe-Gullen was immediately appointed Demonstrator of Anatomy, while at Kingston, where there were no women graduates yet, six women sat on the Board of Trustees. Not surprisingly, one of these women was Dr Trout. Besides contributing most generously to the formation of the College, she had donated a scholarship of fifty dollars a year,[20] quite a large sum in those days, and she was gratefully regarded as the Kingston college's most generous benefactor. The Kingston girls never forgot how much she had done for them.

But Dr Trout was soon to be forgotten in Toronto, for she was approaching the end of her work there. By 1887 her nervous bodily ailments were again exhausting her, and she and Edward moved to Scarborough, to a house they called Gowan Hall. Amelia Tefft went with them, a cheerful companion for Jennie Trout in her seclusion — for though Edward continued to work at the *Monetary Times,* his wife was ready to retire. She was only forty-six, but she was not at all well, and in any case she had already done more than one lifetime's work. She had fought the good fight faithfully, if somewhat unwillingly, so surely she should now be allowed to remove herself from society and the publicity that she had never really relished.

Dr Trout had never been a keen fighter. Although she had been prepared to fight when the cause required it and her beliefs demanded it, she was not such an aggressive campaigner as Emily Stowe. Nor did she have the staying power. In her rivalry with the Stowes, it was she who lost out: in effect, she lost the medical school skirmish simply because the Stowes got their college too — and in 1895, when the two colleges amalgamated, it was the Kingston college that closed down and moved its students to Toronto. Yes, she lost that fight. Eventually she even lost her reputation to Emily Stowe — the reputation of being Canada's first qualified woman doctor.

She may not have minded in either case, for her ambition wasn't a personal ambition. She fought for principles and justice, not for herself, and this shows very clearly in her portraits. Although pictures of Dr Trout in middle life show a very firm chin, the face is gentle and rather thoughtful. It is not the face of a woman who has to be top. Nor does it have the pugnacity of Dr Stowe's pictures. Some of Dr Stowe's portraits look so very fierce and show such bulldog determination that one wonders how any male ever had the courage to say 'no' to her.

This, too, may explain why Emily Stowe has been remembered

MEDICAL EDUCATION FOR WOMEN IN ONTARIO

1880-1906

KINGSTON

QUEEN'S UNIVERSITY
FACULTY OF MEDICINE

TORONTO

UNIVERSITY OF TORONTO
FACULTY OF MEDICINE

Royal College of Physicians and Surgeons, Kingston, known as the Royal College (affiliated with Queen's)

April 1880
Queen's summer MEDICAL COURSE FOR WOMEN begins

Oct. 1881. Students from summer course join the regular medical course.

Oct. 1883
WOMEN'S MEDICAL COLLEGE established (affiliated with Queen's)

1894-95
Women's Medical College closes and its students are absorbed in the Toronto Women's Medical College, which changes its name to the ONTARIO MEDICAL COLLEGE FOR WOMEN

1892
Royal College unites with Queen's College

1879-1883
Augusta Stowe (Victoria College) studies at Toronto School of Medicine.

1887
Toronto School of Medicine becomes University of Toronto Faculty of Medicine

1903
Trinity Medical School joins University of Toronto Faculty of Medicine

Oct. 1883
WOMAN'S MEDICAL COLLEGE established (affiliated with University of Trinity College and University of Toronto)

1906
Ontario Medical College for Women closes and its students are absorbed in University of Toronto Faculty of Medicine

Neither women's college was empowered to grant degrees so students sat the exams of the affiliated universities: Kingston students graduated MD CM, Queen's; Toronto students graduated MD CM, Trinity; MB, Toronto: MD CM, Victoria. After 1895, students of the Ontario Medical College for Women could sit the exams of any university they chose.

while Jennie Trout has not. You couldn't be in a room with Dr Stowe and not be aware of it. But Dr Trout . . . . Who on earth was she? That quiet old lady who poured the tea? Really? What was she doctor *of*?

As Jennie Trout grew older, many people may have met her without knowing of or valuing her medical career, for she came to take more interest in Christianity and missions than in medicine. This doesn't mean that she ever forgot she was a doctor — far from it. She was always ready to minister to her neighbours or to advise her family to take plentiful exercise as a means of retaining their health. But she no longer ran a regular practice.

This resulted in a curious situation which again contrasts with Emily Stowe's. Dr Stowe had produced her family *before* studying medicine. Dr Trout had her family after she retired from it.[21] She and Edward had no children of their own, but they adopted a couple of Jennie's relatives: she was their great-aunt before she became their mother.

In spite of her ill health, Jennie Trout lived to be an octogenarian, and her final years were passed in Los Angeles, worrying a little about Edward's health — which wasn't as robust as it used to be — but mostly occupying herself contentedly with church and family affairs: writing a few letters, contributing to missions, reading her Bible.

As she sat there, in the warm Los Angeles sun, so quietly reading her Bible, did she ever think back to her active pioneering days in a colder climate? It was all a long way off in space as well as time, and she had no Augusta to keep her in touch with the latest victories. No Augusta to carry on the fight for her. But there was Elizabeth Smith-Shortt.

Elizabeth wasn't a daughter, but she had been a form of disciple of Dr Trout — Elizabeth Smith, gallant girl graduate of Kingston. When Dr Trout had encouraged Elizabeth to go to Queen's she had never thought that the young girl would have to suffer the same sort of experience that she had had at the Toronto School of Medicine. In fact it had been precisely to avoid such an experience that Dr Trout had encouraged the girl to take the Queen's course.

ONTARIO MEDICAL COLLEGE
FOR WOMEN

When the college closed in 1906, it had eleven women on its staff:

Ann Augusta Stowe-Gullen (MD Victoria, 1883; MD CM Trinity), Professor of Diseases of Children.

Lelia Ada Davis (MB Toronto, 1889; MD CM Trinity), Demonstrator of Pathology.

Jennie Gray (MD CM Trinity, 1892), Associate Professor of Gynaecology. (Later Mrs Wildman.)

Ida Eliza Lynd (MD CM Trinity, 1890), Lecturer in Materia Medica.

Emma Leila Skinner (MB Toronto, 1896; MD CM Trinity), Lecturer in Obstetrics. (Later Mrs Gordon.)

Rowena Grace Douglas Hume (MD CM Trinity, 1899), Lecturer in Bacteriology.

Minerva Margaret Greenaway (MD CM Trinity, 1899), Lecturer in Diseases of Children.

Jean McDonald Willson (MB Toronto, 1897), Lecturer in Medical Psychology.

Helen MacMurchy (MB Toronto, 1900; MD Toronto, 1901), Lecturer in Medicine.

Eleanor Lucas (MD CM Trinity, 1903), Assistant in Anatomy. (Later Mrs Bennett.)

Isabella Smith Wood (MD CM Trinity, 1902), Assistant in Anatomy.

IDA LYND (Trinity, 1890)
Born at Bondhead, in 1857, Dr Lynd was educated at Hamilton Ladies College and at the Woman's Medical College in Toronto. After graduation, she served on the staff of the college and was also one of the first staff members of the Women's College Hospital. She died in 1943.

JENNIE GRAY WILDMAN (Trinity, 1892)
Jennie Gray (Mrs Wildman) was born in Dundas. With Dr Lynd, she took charge of the first clinics run by the Ontario Medical College for Women. These clinics were the forerunner of the Women's Dispensary, which grew to become the Women's College Hospital, and Dr Wildman played an active role in all three stages of the hospital's development. She moved to Barrie in 1928 and died there, in 1953, at the age of 90.

EMMA SKINNER GORDON (Toronto, 1896)
Another staff member of the Ontario Medical College for Women, Emma

Skinner (Mrs Gordon) was on the staff of the Women's Dispensary and the Women's College Hospital. In addition, she was well known for her welfare work, running a club for boys, founding the Merton St. Gospel Mission and campaigning for the Woman's Christian Temperance Union. She died in 1949, aged 89.

ROWENA DOUGLAS HUME (Trinity, 1899)

Dr Hume took postgraduate studies in the United States and England before returning to Canada to take a staff position at the Ontario Medical College for Women. For many years she was Chief of Obstetrics at the Women's College Hospital. After retiring from the hospital, she ran a private practice. This was still occupying her when, at the age of 89, she was attacked and murdered by a transient worker — one of the unemployed whom Dr Hume was in the habit of helping by paying them to do odd jobs around her house.

4

Freshwomen at Queen's

ELIZABETH SMITH was of the same metal as the other pioneer women doctors, and before beginning to study medicine, she had come to terms with the thought that 'what did not hurt Mrs Jennie Trout would not hurt us'.[1] But this was only a thought, a resolve that if the worst came to the worst, by goodness, she would stick it out too. And it was a hypothetical resolve, because the auspices were so promising that it didn't look as if she was going to have to face any problems more serious than passing her exams.

When Elizabeth set out on the road to become a doctor, she had male as well as female support. This was partly because of her character. She was a self-assured, pretty girl with natural wit and charm, and men found themselves helping her, not because she fought them into the ground, but simply because they liked her. They also admired her: for all her prettiness, her intentions were obviously serious.

She was almost the same age as Augusta, only two years younger, but her background had been very different. Her parents, Sylvester and Damaris Smith, lived at Mountain Hall in Winona.[2] There Elizabeth had been educated by a private governess, before being sent to Winona School and, later, to the Hamilton Collegiate Institute. While Augusta had been brought up in a campaigning atmosphere where you fought for every privilege and struggled for every penny, Elizabeth's early life had been far less tempestuous. In later years, she was to become as active a suffragette as Augusta, but as a young girl she felt no driving urge to fight 'male man' for her privileges: male man had always been rather kind to her, and besides, a certain number of privileges had come to her naturally, simply because she was an intelligent and attractive child of a well-to-do family.

Elizabeth knew, for instance, that her parents could afford her college fees. And if she had to go to the States to study, then that wouldn't strain their budget either. Her parents were quite prepared to follow Jennie Trout's first suggestion and send Elizabeth to Ann Arbor in Michigan, if that were the most comfortable and the best way for their daughter to graduate — and it looked as if it might be, since in the 1870's, when Elizabeth was first making enquiries about medical schools, there were no facilities for women in Canada.

But changes were under way by 1879, when Elizabeth took the matriculation exam of the Council of the College of Physicians and Surgeons (her first step towards studying medicine). Eighteen seventy-nine was the year Queen's decided that, in future, it would take a few women — and one of Elizabeth's matriculation examiners was from Kingston. He was Mr Knight, a 'capital man' who was impressed by young Miss Smith and told her that Queen's Medical Faculty was prepared to start a special summer course for women, provided there were sufficient applicants to make it worth while.

Two other girls were present at the matriculation exams.[3] One was Augusta Stowe, who was up for the second time, having failed maths on her first attempt, and the other was a delicate young girl called Emma Parmenter — one of Dr Trout's protegées, who seems to have had a firm spirit but failing health. Poor Miss Parmenter was very nervous, and didn't pass, but both Augusta and Elizabeth came through with flying colours. Augusta was already looking to Victoria as a possible place to study, but Elizabeth came away determined to follow up the Queen's offer.

As soon as she returned home, she set to work to gather in the medical girls. She wrote to Queen's to learn more of the project, she wrote to Augusta Stowe to try and enlist her help, she wrote to anyone she thought might be interested, and in July she put an announcement in *The Globe,* stating that 'Ladies wishing to study medicine in Canada will hear of something to their advantage by communicating with Box 31, Winona.' One of the first people to write to Box 31 was Augusta Stowe, who said that she would indeed be 'glad to hear of anything that will be of advantage to me as a Medical Student.'[4] But in fact Augusta didn't feel that the Queen's course would be of advantage to her. Her mother had already explained why, in a personal letter to Elizabeth:

In the first place, another year would be too long for her to wait, and there is every objection to summer courses. No person can study as well then as in cold weather, you cannot dissect, and by the profession generally they would never be recognized as of equal value with the winter courses. There is never the same hospital advantages in summer as winter. With regard to the excessive value of a Canadian degree, it is more imaginary than real, and if obtained from separate or summer courses its value would fall.[5]

Other replies were equally discouraging. One said:

Don't be in a hurry to teach Ladies the 'curious arts' Acts (xix. 19) of sorcery and witchcraft called in scripture Pharmacies upon which Pharmacy is based, get instructed yourself in the greatest revolution in physiology and Materia Medica, known as the Gospel Health Movement.
> Yours in the Great Physician Jesus the Christ,
> Victor B. Hall.[6]

Fortunately, eleven of the letters did express serious interest in the project and this was more than enough to get it moving. As the months went by, the number dropped to ten . . . to nine . . . to seven . . . as the various parents found they couldn't afford to educate a daughter as well as a son, but Queen's had committed itself. Even if only three students presented themselves for the summer course, it would be worth the trouble, for Queen's was aware that it was making history. The medical course for women, which was due to open in April, 1880, was going to be the first of its kind ever given in Canada.

It started very pleasantly. When Elizabeth arrived in Kingston, she was welcomed most cordially by the professors, four of whom had given up their summer holidays especially to take on the girls. They made her feel all the more welcome by affecting delighted

surprise at her youth and modesty. They had, one of them explained, expected that Miss Smith, Organizer, would be a 'dried
up old maid'. Elizabeth blushed demurely, and then quickly wrote
home to her family telling them of her flattering reception — and
also telling them not to turn up their eyes and cough sceptically:
she was *trying* to be demure and modest!

In the midst of all this demureness, she was rustling round
Kingston, booking herself into a boarding house where one of the
other women was staying ($2.50 a week), buying a copy of *Gray's
Anatomy* ($6.50), paying her registration fee ($2.00) and also buy-
ing four notebooks, a box of surgical tools, four knives, a hook, a
pair of scissors and two forceps (total $3.00). Even if her father
did have money, it was being very carefully spent.

Soon Elizabeth was making friends with the two other students, Alice Skimmen McGillivray and Elizabeth Robb Beatty.
Mrs McGillivray and her husband had already established themselves in the boarding house — a good choice of lodging since the
owner's son had just taken his MD and was willing to lend the
women students his books and bones. Elizabeth liked Mrs
McGillivray immediately: she was so bright and sprightly. Alice
McGillivray was about nineteen years old at the time and had been
married more than a year. Elizabeth described her as a 'piquant,
jolly little brick' but 'thoroughly womanly and sensible'.

She also regarded Miss Beatty as a 'brick', but not quite such a
jolly one. Miss Beatty was older than the other two, of a more
serious temperament — she had already decided to be a missionary
— and apparently she looked as if she was ready to die in harness.
Elizabeth cast her in the role of 'old maid', the role she herself was
so glad *not* to have been cast in by the professors: 'I tell you, there's
the girl that would make a noble wife — but she's a man hater.
She's a master of sarcasm, a wrestler in argument, possesses a fund
of wit, quiet, steady, true, would go through a mountain rather
than go round it.'[7]

Elizabeth Smith didn't know Elizabeth Beatty very well when she
wrote this description and it sounds slightly forced when compared
with her spontaneous praise of sprightly Mrs McGillivray. But
Elizabeth was to become very fond of the future missionary. One
couldn't help liking Miss Beatty. She had such a dry wit and such
a pithy turn of phrase that one apt sentence from her could make

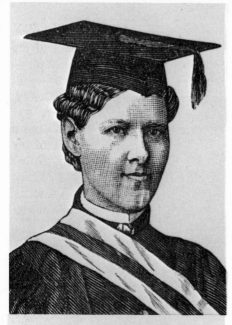

Dr Elizabeth Beatty (left)

Dr Elizabeth Smith-Shortt (below left)

Dr Alice McGillivray (below right)

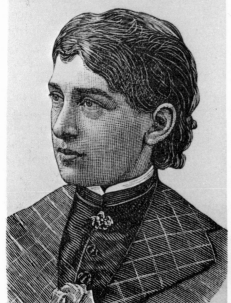

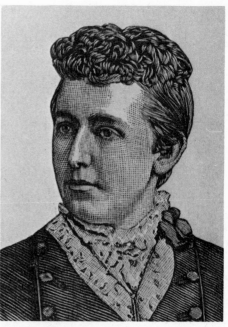

the other two girls helpless with laughter, even at the gloomiest times.

They were an unlikely threesome, each with a different temperament, but all feminists at heart and all determined to get those two letters: MD. They stood their first year very well, bracing themselves to witness their first operation, to take their first dissection class, to observe the gruesome treatment which had to be given to some of the patients at the lunatic asylum and the hospital. As Dr Stowe had predicted, dissecting corpses was not a pleasant occupation in hot weather. Most of the dissection was done before the summer really heated up, but even so the odours were appalling and the three stalwart maidens seem to have spent most of the classes trying to appear stalwart and desperately hoping that they weren't going to be sick. They were determined to be as unmoved as they imagined young men to be. Frailty, thy name was *not* going to be woman.

As a matter of fact, they were getting through their course far more competently than the normal male first year students. With delighted enthusiasm, the professors praised the girls, but they were a little appalled at the speed with which these pupils were learning. The professors were used to teaching carefree young men who spent as much time playing as working during their first year. But these girls never stopped working. Some days their classes ran from eight in the morning till seven in the evening — and still they put in a good four hours studying before going to bed. They were doing too *much* work!

The professors persuaded the young ladies to take a brief holiday in mid-session. It was a welcome break for everyone although the girls would rather have gone on working. There was so much to learn — and they so dearly wanted to excel. Elizabeth was planning to study during much of the winter, and Alice McGillivray was planning to join the men's chemistry course when the University officially opened in October — it was now possible for a woman to do so.

In the autumn of 1880, Queen's would be taking women for the first time in its regular classes (a result of the 1879 decision on co-education). There would just be a handful of girls at first, some of whom would be studying Arts, but it did mean that the university was now fully open to women. This being the case, Elizabeth asked the Registrar if her trio could sign on for second year medicine in October — instead of having to wait for the resumption of their special course the next spring. But the Registrar decided that this wouldn't do: when it came to medicine, there was still that modesty problem.

However, the Registrar's reply turned out to be a delayed Yes, rather than a No. Since only two new women students were interested in attending the second session of the women's medical course it was decided not to continue it and, in October, 1881, the girls joined the men's class. This meant that they lost a year's studies, which caused them considerable annoyance — and also caused them to graduate one year after Augusta Stowe. Emily Stowe had been wise to reject the Queen's course.

Nevertheless, conditions were made very pleasant for the women at Queen's. They were provided with a separate dissecting room and a separate cloakroom and waiting room — and, for awkward lectures, like obstetrics and medical jurisprudence, they sat in a little room adjacent to the general classroom so that any embarrassed blushes would go unnoticed by the young men. For their part, the male students behaved extremely well. When the first women had entered Queen's the previous year, their arrival hadn't sparked any resentment. If one can judge from the attitude of the *Queen's College Journal,* the women were actually welcomed — even if the welcome was slightly patronizing:

FRESHWOMEN — We were standing in the Hall on Wednesday waiting for something to turn up for incorporation in this issue, when the door of the ante-room over the entrance opened and on it came — we can't help it if our readers do not believe us; but we assure them on the word of the editor that it is a fact — a flock of a-a-a-freshwomen, I suppose we must call them. We were utterly dumbfounded. Where in the name of Minerva did they come from? But before we had recovered our normal equanimity they came up and asked the locality of a certain class-room. We blushed and pointed vacantly down the corridor and then vanished. We have now completely recovered from the shock, and extend to the young ladies our most cordial welcome, and hope that they are only the first installment of a large number yet to come. The more the merrier.[8]

Elizabeth enjoyed being part of the university. Even during the summer session, she had been courted competitively by the young men of Kingston, but now she was really under siege. She was known by the students as 'the pretty one', but she might just as well have been called 'the eligible one'. Alice McGillivray was married, Elizabeth Beatty said she didn't like men, and the three additional women who had joined the medical course were not really girl-friend material. There was Helen Reynolds, who was large, and rather reserved in those days: 'one of the saucy independent kind and stands up to an immense height on her dignity.'⁹ There was Margaret Corliss who was not only married, but very old — at least forty-two! And there was Annie Dickson. Annie Dickson was a pro-fessor's daughter who had attended part of the summer session and was studying full-time now. She wasn't at all popular. She was prim and self-sacrificing and 'too good for human nature's daily food.'¹⁰ Elizabeth, on the other hand, was just the food that most of the students wanted.

But she wouldn't allow them more than a nibble. She had come to Kingston to get her degree and nothing was going to deflect her from it. Besides, she was intensely interested in her work. Although she felt she was an old hand at medicine by this time and was no longer overawed by the great weight of knowledge that faced her, she still felt that medicine was the most worthy calling in the world. First and foremost, she wanted to be a doctor.

It looked as if she would become one with ease, and without any opposition: by the end of the 1881-82 session, both staff and students were complimenting each other on the success of this experiment in medical co-education. It just showed what could be done if people behaved sensibly. Very true. But unfortunately the most respon-sible students graduated at the end of the session, and in the fall their seats were filled by a distinctly irresponsible group of fresh-men.

The session began badly and by November most of the students were being as ribald as the freshmen. Strangely enough, it was not the obstetrics class that the girls came to dread most. Although this offered the easiest opportunity to make embarrassing jokes, the obstetrics lectures were given by the Dean, who stood no nonsense from the young men and had no objections to the young ladies.

But the physiology lectures became a form of torture. Dr Fen-wick, the physiology lecturer, had been pleasant and easy the pre-

vious year, but he had had some disagreement with the Faculty
and had decided to take it out on the women — possibly because the
Faculty supported the women. Whatever the cause, he had done
a complete *volte-face* and was now saying that 'he had no respect
for women who studied medicine, and would not have them in his
house.'[11] As he was obliged to have them in his classroom, he made
the most of it, giving the students every opportunity to be lewd and
rude and crude, and producing quite a number of lewdities himself.
And of course it was pervasive. Although other classes were conducted in a more kindly and orderly manner, the student atmosphere had changed. The women had become scapegoats.

By this time, the two Elizabeths and Alice McGillivray were calling themselves Shadrach, Meshach and Abednego — because they
were going through fire! — and poor Helen Reynolds, in spite of her
'saucy independence' had become so upset that it was making her
ill. But at least the Queen's women had each other for company.
They didn't have to face the male onslaught alone as Augusta Stowe
was doing. And they did have most of the staff on their side. They
also had an ally in the janitor, Tom Coffee, who would let them
into the classrooms first, so that they wouldn't have to walk in
through a barrage of sniggers, whispers and, occasionally, booby
traps. 'Yeese can be goin' in now leddies,' he would inform the girls,
before going off to ring the bell that would summon the young
men.[12] By the time the men poured into the classroom, the young
ladies were demurely, and safely, settled in their seats.

And they fought back. When, for the umpteenth time, the offensive Dr Fenwick leered at the students, and said, 'This reminds me
of an anecdote . . .' the young ladies rose in a body, walked quietly
out of the classroom, and went straight to the Registrar's office. The
Registrar was a kindly man, and he tried to settle the matter amic-
ably, calming the young ladies and reasoning with the young men.
But he didn't succeed because while he was still trying to smooth
over the whole affair and unruffle all the feathers, a letter appeared
in the newspapers, presenting the men's viewpoint, and the whole
affair became public.

Soon Dr Fenwick was also talking to the Press[13] maintaining that
he had said nothing offensive and that anyway he had to garble
his lectures when ladies attended them. This became the main platform of the male students: that, since women had been present, the

more embarrassing subjects were not being taught in sufficient detail. The men weren't learning what they should be learning, and they weren't getting their money's worth. It wasn't true, but it sounded convincing, and it became the men's battle cry.

By this time the dispute had developed into a full-scale war, possibly the first student revolt to take place in Canada. And it wasn't so very different from recent student riots. It was more orderly, but there was a familiar ring to some of the demands. Although the primary demand was that women should leave the college, the students were also claiming administration rights, saying that since they paid fees to the college, they ought to have a say in its management. Then the students delivered an ultimatum: if the Faculty didn't get rid of the women, the men would leave and move in a body to Trinity Medical School in Toronto.

This threat was too much for the Faculty. Queen's couldn't afford to lose its entire medical school — and it would certainly do so if it didn't back down, because Trinity had agreed to accept the striking medics. Yet how could one turn out these hard-working girls, who had already gone so far towards their degrees?

All along, the city of Kingston had been staunchly supporting the girls, and now a group of prominent citizens, including a number of ex-mayors, managed to bring about a compromise. On their side, the students would be allowed to win their point — no more women would be accepted — but the present women would not be expelled, they would be allowed to stay on at Queen's until they graduated, taking their classes separately from the men.

It was an uneasy compromise, a truce rather than a peace, and both Faculty and women students were therefore relieved when they heard the first rumblings of the move to start a women's college in Toronto. And when the Toronto planners reached a deadlock, because of the disagreement about having women on the staff, and Dr Trout transferred her offer to Kingston — why, naturally, she was welcomed with as much enthusiasm as gratitude.

Besides, it was most fitting that Queen's should sponsor a women's medical college. Queen's had, after all, provided the first Canadian medical course for women, even if the course hadn't been entirely successful. And now Queen's would be able to fulfil its obligation to these women students and see them through to graduation. It would be able to continue to educate women in medicine.

Theoretically, the women's college would not be part of the university, it would be an affiliated college, and in this it would be no different from Queen's existing medical school which was also an affiliated college. Certainly the students of the Women's Medical College considered themselves to be Queen's students: their College Song mentions 'Old QC' as often as 'WMC'. And it also mentions 'Prof. McG.'

Alice McGillivray was appointed to the staff immediately on her graduation. She and the two Elizabeths were in their last year of medicine during the medical college's first year of life and, when they graduated in 1884, she was the only possible staff member. Dr Beatty was bound for India, and Dr Smith had gone off to Hamilton to set up a practice there. But in any case, Dr McGillivray would have been an obvious choice. She had been an exceptional student, a gold medalist, and before long she was promoted to Professor of Obstetrics and Diseases of Women and Children, a position she held until she and her husband moved to Chicago in 1889.[14]

Three years after her appointment, she was joined on the staff by Elizabeth Smith, who had married one of her Kingston boyfriends — Adam Shortt, the future Professor of Political Economy — and returned to live in the city. As Dr Smith-Shortt, Elizabeth was appointed Professor of Medical Jurisprudence and Sanitary Science — a position which, strangely, had been held by Dr Fenwick (the troublesome lecturer) until Elizabeth took over.

Each year from then on the number of female staff members grew, as did the number of students. But, little by little, the college lost ground to its sister college in Toronto. Although the Kingston college could list quite a few Local Advantages in its annual calendar, although it could offer facilities for the students at the Penitentiary, the Gaol, the General Hospital and the Hotel Dieu, and although it could announce that Kingston 'is a most orderly city. A lady can walk the streets at all hours without meeting any disrespect. . . .'[15] even so, Toronto had many more Local Advantages. Besides claiming to be one of the healthiest places on the continent, Toronto could offer its medical students a far greater selection of hospitals and clinics, and it could even offer future missionaries a special course in theology at Knox College. After all, Toronto was the provincial capital, the centre where just about everything was happening. And it was growing rapidly. So when the authorities came to their senses and admitted that they didn't need two women's medical colleges, it was inevitable that it would be the Kingston college which closed down.

This happened in 1894-95. Toronto Woman's Medical College changed its name to the Ontario Medical College for Women, the Kingston students moved to Toronto, the staff didn't (there was no place for them: Toronto already had six lady staff members), and the Kingston Women's Medical College faded into history. But it had left its mark. During its brief span of life, the college had graduated over thirty doctors and many of them were to be heard of in the future.

The most famous was probably Elizabeth Smith-Shortt, the pioneer of the Queen's course. Her husband, the distinguished historian and political economist, Professor Adam Shortt, CGM, was one of Canada's academic giants, but Elizabeth didn't rise to fame on his coat-tails. As a professor in her early twenties she was already making a name for herself and getting immortalized in a college song ('O Doctor, Cut my leg off, Shortt, Shortt, Shortt'[16]), and although she acted as hostess for her husband and foster-mother to his students, she was very active in her own field too. She taught, wrote medical papers, gave speeches, founded the Queen's Alumnae Society, sponsored Kingston's musical club, established one of the first YWCA's, started a local Council of Women, and also gave birth to a few children.

When her husband became Civil Service Commissioner in Ottawa, the tempo increased. Her energy was formidable. When one reads any of the eulogies which were written about Dr Smith-Shortt, one's first reaction is: 'How did she fit it all in?' She lived till her ninetieth year, but even so the sum total of her achievements is staggering. She helped to form the Victorian Order of Nurses *and* the Women's Canadian Club. For years she was Vice-President of Ontario's Council of Women, she acted successively as National Convener of Immigration, of Public Health and of Mental Hygiene, she was the first head of Ontario's Mother's Allowances Board. . . . She never stopped! One moment she was fighting the National Dairy Council for the acceptance of oleomargarine, the next moment she was campaigning for illegitimate children to be registered as legitimate if their parents married. Or else she was founding a home for aged gentlewomen — the Elizabeth Residence, named in her honour. Look at almost anything connected with women, welfare or medicine, and there is Dr Elizabeth Smith-Shortt in the thick of it, bristling with energy and relieving the seriousness of her work with bright stabs of wit, some of which sound as if they could have been spoken by pithy Miss Beatty. 'That woman's head is as untidy inside as out,' she said of one of her antagonists. Of another, a cabinet minister who was making a long evasive speech, she said, 'He is there by geography, not by ability.' Even in her old age, when she was frail and ill, she could still be lightheartedly witty, and although both sight and hearing began to fail, her perception remained as clear as it had been in those college days when she was writing her parents thumbnail sketches of her student friends.

And what of them, her fellow students, sprightly Mrs McG and caustic Miss B?

Alice McGillivray, the first female professor at the Kingston Women's Medical College, had moved to Chicago, but she was back in Canada within ten years, practising in Hamilton with her husband, who also became a doctor. Their practice seems to have been more successful than their marriage, for Alice's husband developed a passion for birds and filled the house with live pheasants which would flit around the rooms, perching at random on piano and visitors. This became too much for Alice, who liked everything to be spic and span, and she moved out to live with her sister Nellie Skimmen, who had followed her into medicine and had also set up a practice in Hamilton (Nellie had been a student at Kingston when Alice was a professor). So husband and wife lived separately, but they continued to work together. On at least one occasion they performed an operation together — a trifle worrying for the patient perhaps.

Alice McGillivray died before she was sixty,[17] but her classmate, Elizabeth Beatty, lived into her eighties — keeping up the longevity average of the early women doctors. As she had intended, she became a missionary, and in 1884 she set off for India as the Presbyterian Church of Canada's first woman missionary doctor.[18] She travelled out with Lady Dufferin, a 'sympathetic and congenial voyager' who became a staunch supporter of her medical work. Dr Beatty's work was with the Indians, not with the British, so when she arrived at Indore in Central India, she moved beyond the

British Residency and rented herself a mud house, using the lower floor as a dispensary and the upper as a four-bed hospital. She then set out to make herself sympathetic and congenial to the Indians, learning Hindi as fast as she could, administering to the sick, and training Indian women as nurses.

It has been said that Dr Beatty was 'most original in her methods of approach to the people' and that she was a 'woman of strong personality', so it looks as if her quick wit and dry humour stood her in good stead when she found herself virtually alone in the field. She seems to have been very popular. She was consulted by the rich as well as the poor, and the Maharani of Indore was so impressed by Dr Beatty that she gave her some land on which to build a special hospital for women. This was the first women's hospital in Central India.

Unfortunately, Dr Beatty did not see the hospital completed. After only six years in Indore, her health broke down and she had to return to Canada. Only six years, yet during those years Dr Beatty had laid the foundations of what was to become one of Canada's greatest medical missions. Many women doctors were to follow her to Indore, some from the Kingston college and some from the Toronto one, but it was dry-humoured Dr Beatty in her mud-hut dispensary who led the way.

Between them, the Toronto and Kingston colleges trained so many missionary doctors and so many other doctors too that it is easy to imagine that the story of Canada's early medical women was confined to Ontario. But all these women did not necessarily come from Ontario. Some were Winnipeg girls, others were Montrealers or Maritimers. And a good many of them returned to their native province to practise.

When they arrived home to hang up their shingles, they were seldom considered the pioneers, for they were the second wave, the younger generation, the girls who had been born late enough to graduate in Canada. Although Ontario was the home of our first women's medical colleges and the home of our first women doctors, the other provinces had their pioneers too, graduates from the United States. And they were often only a step behind Doctors Stowe and Trout. Here, as early as 1876, is Dr Charlotte Whitehead Ross running a practice for women and children in Montreal. Here she is again, a few years later, busy setting bones and sewing up wounds on a lumber camp in Whitemouth, Manitoba. Here, in Winnipeg are Dr Amelia Yeomans and her daughter Dr Lilian Yeomans, both graduates from Ann Arbor, Michigan, both well established by 1885. Here, in New Brunswick, is Elizabeth Secord, licensed to practise as early as 1883. And here in Halifax is Dr Maria Angwin, an 1882 graduate.

Women doctors were sprouting like wild flowers, even while such young girls as Elizabeth Smith and Augusta Stowe were only starting their medical training.

VERSES FROM THE *QUEEN'S COLLEGE GIRLS' SONG, 1886*
(Tune — *Funicoli funicola*)

We are a hearty band of working lasses,
    In Old Q.C.! in old Q.C.!
And now we find relief from all our classes,
    In drinking tea! in drinking tea!
'Tis here we talk of our *Association,*
    So kind and free! so kind and free!
To all who care to join of any nation,
    Or far countree! or far countree!

Chorus: Joy then! joy then! joy to old Q.C.
          Love and peace and all prosperitie!
          We like its ways, its work, its Profs., its boys,
            but mostly the *degree,*
          Which *all* of us are sure to take before we
          leave Q.C.

And if our nerves we have too much been trying,
    In old Q.C.! in old Q.C.!
And on our couch in *solemn* state are lying,
    W.M.C.! W.M.C.!
We cry, and very soon our sisters hear us,
    One soon we see! one soon we see!
With pills and tonics rapidly she cures us
    Dear Prof. McG—! dear Prof. McG—!

Chorus: Joy then! joy then! etc.

But oh! the joy and bliss of Convocation,
    At old Q.C.! at old Q.C.!
Just think! there's not e'en *one* examination,
    For me! for me! rejoice with me!
We *now* can spend our days in learned chatter,
    Of old Q.C.! of old Q.C.!
We may get married! but that is no matter,
    We've a *degree*! we've a *degree*!

Chorus: Joy then! joy then! etc.

SIX GRADUATES OF THE KINGSTON
WOMEN'S MEDICAL COLLEGE

HELEN ELIZABETH REYNOLDS RYAN
(MD CM Queen's, 1885)
Helen Elizabeth Reynolds — the large and rather reserved girl who was at
college with Elizabeth Smith — made a success of her life in three different
fields: as a doctor, as a suffragette and as a wife and mother. She was the first
woman to be granted membership to the Canadian Medical Association, and
she carried on a practice until 1907 — at first working with her brother in
Mount Forest and then, after her marriage, running an extensive practice in
Sudbury, Ont. She married Thomas John Ryan and had five children, and she
and her family moved to Victoria in 1907. In Victoria, she joined the local
Council of Women and became very active in the franchise movement,
travelling round British Columbia lecturing and drumming up support for the
movement. She died in Victoria in 1947 at the age of 87.

ISOBEL McCONVILLE
(MD CM Queen's, 1889)
worked in Kingston for many years, at the Hotel Dieu Hospital and as
physician to the sisters both at the Hotel Dieu and at Notre Dame Convent.

ELLA BLAYLOCK ATHERTON
(MD CM Queen's, 1887)
Ella Blaylock (Mrs Atherton) won a wide reputation as a surgeon and is said
to have been the first woman to practise abdominal surgery in New Hampshire.
Her husband was American and she practised for 44 years in the United
States, where she became a founder and trustee of the Nassau Memorial
Hospital. Although Dr Atherton lived most of her life in the States,
she was not American by origin: she was born in Lancashire, England, and
brought up and educated in Canada, studying at McGill before she went to the
Women's Medical College at Kingston.

CLARA DEMOREST
(MD CM Queen's, 1890)
was one of the first women to practise in Alberta. She set up a practice in
Calgary in 1905.

AGNES DOUGLAS CRAINE
(MD CM Queen's, 1888)
A descendant of the first settlers to land at Chateauguay, Quebec, Dr Craine repaid Queen's University very handsomely for the privilege of being allowed to study medicine. During her life, she contributed (anonymously) nearly $400,000 to the university. This fantastically generous donation was made to further the work of biochemistry, and part of the fund was used to establish the Craine Chair of Biochemistry and the Craine Building at Queen's. Apart from her student years at Kingston and postgraduate study in Europe, Dr Craine spent her life at Smith's Falls, Ontario. There she was born, there she practised and there, in 1937, she died, at the age of 75 years.

WILHELMINA FRASER STUART
(MD CM Queen's, 1890)
Wilhelmina Fraser (Mrs Stuart) went to India as a missionary, serving at Ratlam and Mhow.

FIVE INDORE DOCTORS

MARION OLIVER
(MD CM Queen's, 1886)
Marion Oliver joined Elizabeth Beatty at Indore in 1887 and spent her life
there building up the mission. She died in Canada in 1913 only a year after
her retirement.

MARGARET MacKELLAR
(MD CM Queen's, 1890)
Margaret MacKellar was a medical missionary in India for 40 years, first at
Indore and then in Neemuch, Central India, where she was the pioneering
doctor, and where she set up the first hospital. For many years she served as
secretary and then as chairman of the Christian Medical College for Women,
which was established at Ludhiana in the Punjab, and during the First War
she was attached to the RAMC at the Freeman Thomas Hospital in Bombay.
She was awarded the Kaisar-i-Hind medal for her years of service in India
and, in 1929, she was awarded an honorary LL D by Queen's University.

Born in Mull, Scotland, in 1861, Dr MacKellar came to Canada as a child
and attended public school in Bruce County before studying at Queen's.
She died in Toronto in 1941.

AGNES TURNBULL
(MD CM Queen's, 1892)
Agnes Turnbull was also decorated with the Kaisar-i-Hind medal, which was
bestowed on her for her work during a terrible outbreak of plague. She was a
Montrealer by birth, going to Kingston for her medical education. She left
for India immediately after her graduation and she served there as a medical
missionary, at Indore and Neemuch, until her death in 1906.

MARY CHRISTINA BEIN McKAY BUCHANAN
(MD CM Trinity, 1888)
Mary McKay (Mrs Buchanan) was a Maritimer from Pictou County. She went
to India in 1888, married there the following year, and died there in 1935.
Although she suffered from ill health most of her years in India, and although
she saw her first child die there at the age of three, she was devoted to the
country, serving as mother, teacher and friend, as well as doctor.

BELLE CHONE OLIVER

(MB Toronto, 1900)

Dr Oliver served at the women's hospitals in Indore, Dhar and Neemuch and in 1915 she was appointed the first medical missionary to Banswara. She was actively concerned in the medical education of Indians, and in 1933 she was appointed Secretary of the Christian Medical Association of India. She died at Fort William in 1947.

5

'Mrs Doctor', East and West

IN 1883, when Dr Maria Angwin was interviewed by the Halifax *Morning Herald,* she stated that there were seven or eight Nova Scotian ladies already practising medicine. Lady doctors were no novelty, she insisted. Why, at least sixty had already graduated from the Woman's Medical College of the New York Infirmary, where she had received her MD the previous year, and the Philadelphia college turned out about thirty graduates each year.

'They are very successful,' Dr Angwin told the reporter. 'They are scattered all through the states, have large expectations and are all doing well.'[1]

Unfortunately, most of the Nova Scotians were also scattered through the States, including the province's first woman graduate in medicine. She was Annie Maxwell Fulton, a Pictou County girl who had graduated from the Woman's Medical College of Pennsylvania in 1873 — preceding even Jennie Trout. But Dr Fulton never practised in Canada. She worked in the United States, married there and died there, at the early age of forty-one.

Maria Angwin also worked in the United States for a while — she spent a year at the New England Hospital before returning to Canada — but she returned home because she felt that Halifax needed a woman doctor. And she intended to be that woman, even if the *Herald's* reporter was sceptical about her chances of success. He seems to have been unpleasantly antagonistic. Surely, he said, it wouldn't be easy for a woman to establish a practice in Halifax. The city's male physicians would be certain to boycott her. After all,

Haligonians hadn't had a woman doctor before, and they did have the reputation of being rather conservative.

The reporter made the most of his interview, using such headlines as 'Sensations in the Dissecting Room' and 'Hacking the Human Form Divine', but there was nothing sensational about Dr Angwin's statements. The more provocative the questions, the more firmly she answered them, and — one suspects — the more angry she became.

'The motto that will hang in my office,' she said, 'is this: if God be for us, who can be against us?'

So much for the reporter. *And* for anyone who would dare to boycott. She then added her punch line:

'If I get a practice in Halifax, I shall stay. If not, I shall go where I can get one, for there are other cities on the continent besides Halifax.'

This challenge to Halifax pride could easily be seen as the reason why Maria Angwin did find a practice in the city, did get licensed, did become accepted by those conservative Haligonians. But in fact the Haligonians weren't as conservative as they were made out to be. As early as 1881, Dalhousie had passed a regulation allowing women to be admitted to the medical college,[2] and although no women were actually enrolled for some years (the first woman MD didn't graduate until 1894), even so, this action showed that Halifax was moving with the times — and moving ahead of many other cities.

Its first lady doctor was also ahead of her time. Dr Angwin wore her hair short which, in the 1880's, was almost as unusual as being a female physician. She was a very definite, no-nonsense type of woman, bold, strong-willed and ready to speak her mind, especially on the evils of alcohol and tobacco. (She was the daughter of a Methodist minister, and strongly opposed to 'stimulants'.)

Maria Angwin lived at her father's house when she first set up her practice,[3] but later she was to move to 52 Spring Garden Road, where she ran her office, and where she lived, together with her sister and a parrot — both of whom gave her great moral support. In spite of her licence, she did meet with a good deal of opposition when she was first working in Halifax, but at least the parrot always recognized her qualifications. 'Somebody wants the doctor,' it would announce throatily each time the doorbell jangled.

Another bell might also be heard in the Angwin household, for Dr Angwin had the novelty of a telephone — which proved to be an inconvenience as much as a convenience. She was frequently called out at night, and off she would go, unchaperoned, even when called to the least reputable parts of town. Foolhardy? What nonsense! She had to go: a patient needed her. Besides, she had a hat pin, didn't she?

In this matter-of-fact and unhesitant manner, Maria Angwin carried on her practice in Halifax for nearly fifteen years, and by the time she died in 1898,[4] she had gone a long way in building the reputation of women as physicians. By this time, Nova Scotia was getting used to lady doctors. Seven more women had joined the profession. Three of them were graduates from New York, but four had done even better than that. They had studied and graduated right here at home, on the campus of Dalhousie University.

Meanwhile, neighbouring New Brunswick wasn't doing at all badly either. It couldn't boast of graduating any women physicians, but it had been licensing them for some years. Back in 1883, Dr Elizabeth Secord had been registered in New Brunswick. She had graduated from Keeokuk, Michigan, and had done postgraduate work in Europe before returning home to open an office at Fredericton Junction.[5]

Elizabeth Secord was the daughter of Daniel Smith of Blissville. She had married a fellow Maritimer, John Secord, had born him one child and had been widowed, all before becoming a medical student. But she seems to have been practising medicine even earlier. She is said to have delivered her sister-in-law's child before she ever became a doctor. This child suffered from 'blackouts' and it was the determination to cure her which prompted Elizabeth Secord to study medicine.[6]

Happily, Dr Secord did succeed in finding a cure for her niece, and she went on to build up a province-wide reputation. She was to practise in New Brunswick for thirty-three years, but not at Fredericton Junction: life became too uncomfortable for her there. Like Maria Angwin, she was adamantly opposed to 'stimulants' and she waged a long and losing battle against a certain Mr Shane, who owned a hotel at Fredericton Junction and who sold liquor in defiance of the law. Dr Secord was determined to get him sent to jail, but Shane had more supporters than she did and it was

Dr Secord who was obliged to leave town. She was not actually run out of town, but she had made too many enemies: it would be easier to start again somewhere else. So she moved to Norton, and then to Farmerston (now Jacksonville) where she succeeded in building up a busy and popular practice. Perhaps she was less aggressive at Farmerston, or perhaps the neighbourhood was more sympathetic to her views. Whatever the case, she didn't retire until a few months before her death in 1916. She was seventy-two years old by then and had been New Brunswick's crusading woman physician since 1883.

Montreal had a woman doctor even earlier, but she wasn't a crusader. She was Charlotte Whitehead Ross,[7] a classmate of Jennie Trout, with whom she had quite a bit in common. Like Dr Trout, Charlotte Ross was extremely religious. And she too was the child of immigrant parents. She had been born in England in 1843,[8] the daughter of Joseph Whitehead, the railway engineer, and she had been brought to Canada at the age of five. Charlotte was also to marry an immigrant, a Scotsman called David Ross.

There are varying stories as to why Charlotte Ross decided to study medicine. She had a sister who was a chronic invalid . . . she had time on her hands in Montreal when her husband was working out West . . . she would need a knowledge of medicine if she was to bring her family to join her husband in the West. . . . Probably all combined to induce her to become a physician. Certainly she started reading medical works when her husband was pioneering in the West and she was left alone with her children in Montreal — feeling bored and unchallenged. She showed such an aptitude for the subject that her family physician lent her his books and encouraged her to go to college. Such talent shouldn't be wasted, he said. She *ought* to become a physician.

Old Mr Whitehead, Charlotte's father, wasn't so enthusiastic. He had not brought up his daughter to be anything so original. She had been given a sheltered and conventional childhood — public school at Clinton, Ontario, and then finishing school at the Sacred Heart Convent in Montreal. And then, of course, marriage. She had married most suitably. David Ross became Whitehead's right-hand man, his aide on the various railway projects. Joseph Whitehead was to land several contracts for railway construction, including the contract to build Section 15 of the new Pacific Railway,[9] and he was to rely heavily on David Ross's ability. A fine young man. The perfect son-in-law.

The contract for Section 15 wasn't awarded until 1877, two years after Charlotte had graduated, but both Ross and Whitehead were busy in the West when she set off for Pennsylvania to study medicine. She therefore felt free to go: she wasn't deserting David. Besides, he supported her studies. If Charlotte became a doctor, then it would be safe to bring the children out West and the family could be together, instead of separated by more than a thousand miles of rough and almost impassable country.

It has been said that Charlotte Ross took ten full years to graduate in medicine, though the Woman's Medical College of Pennsylvania only lists her as a student between 1870 and 1875.[10] Probably she didn't sit any exams during the early years — it certainly sounds as if she was a very 'occasional' student at first. The problem was her family. She was a dutiful mother, wife, sister, daughter, and she put these duties first.

Charlotte already had three children when she enrolled at Philadelphia and she decided to leave them in Montreal. But this wasn't a successful arrangement: she wasn't used to being separated from them as well as from her husband, and she worried about them. Isabel, Minnie and Kate — were they happy without her? Were they being given proper attention? Possibly not. Charlotte returned to Montreal and, the following year, she took her children with her to Pennsylvania. But again her studies were broken off, this time by family tragedies, which compelled her to return home to be a good sister and daughter.

A further handicap was that she returned to Canada — and to her husband — each summer. The consequence of these annual reunions was a series of pregnancies, a depressing and debilitating number of miscarriages, and the birth of a fourth girl, Edith, in 1873. Even when she was sitting her finals, Charlotte was in her almost habitual state of expectancy. Her fifth child and first son was born three months after her graduation. Today, when there is so much talk about how to be a good mother *and* a good career woman, it is interesting to find that there were women facing the same problem a hundred years ago — and eventually succeeding in both spheres.

Charlotte graduated in 1875 (most appropriately writing her

thesis on abortion) and by 1876 she was running a practice for women and children in Montreal.[11] She may even have started to practise in 1875 — the same year as Jennie Trout — but there is no evidence that she was licensed at that time, or that she was ever licensed in Quebec. Her practice was probably very small, easily overlooked by the doyens of the profession. After all, she had not studied medicine in order to serve the public; she had done so specifically to serve her own family, to make it possible for them to live wherever her husband was working.

The plans to join her husband did not bear fruit immediately. In 1878, Charlotte and her mother visited his railway camp and they returned to Montreal convinced that it was no place for children. The two women had lived in tents — that was alright — but the railway workers were not the most suitable influence for young children. They drank heavily and they seemed to attract a rather dubious type of female. The few women that the two wives had noticed in the area didn't seem entirely respectable. In addition, Charlotte and her mother had experienced a plague of grasshoppers when they were out West and had watched in horror while the creatures hopped over the ground, eating every green thing in their path, and sometimes eating bedding and clothing as well. No, this was no place for children.

In 1880, Joseph Whitehead was relieved of his contract with the Canadian Pacific Railway. He had got into difficulties at Cross Lake, where there seemed to be a bottomless marsh. However much fill was poured in to bridge the narrows there, the lake swallowed it and remained as boggy and unstable as ever. It was a losing battle, financially as well as physically, and David Ross, like his father-in-law, was glad to get out of the work. The young man took over a lumber mill, which had belonged to Whitehead, moved it to Whitemouth on the new Pacific Railway, and set it up there on a river that ran through the forest. He then built a log cabin on the bank above the mill and, at last, in 1881, sent for his wife and children.

When Charlotte arrived at Whitemouth, Manitoba, it was not the well-settled farming country that it is today. It was a wild and wooded land, inhabited by the Indian people and by a few lumbermen. The lumbermen were not so very different from the railway workers — in fact some of them were the same men. Mostly young, mostly single, they were tough-living, hard-drinking, hard-working adventurers. All-male, and all men. For the first six months Charlotte was the only white woman in the area. She was also the only doctor. These two attributes worked against each other to place the 'openers of the West' in a totally unexpected dilemma, for they were the type of men who could cope with new territory far more easily than with new ideas. Sophisticates in Toronto might hold literary gatherings to discuss 'the developing role of women', and *The Globe* might record the successes of Dr Stowe or Dr Trout, but out here in the West the idea of a woman being a doctor was inconceivable. It was beyond comprehension, a totally novel concept. And a most dubious one.

Charlotte Whitehead Ross was not a campaigner. She hadn't come west to open male minds to the worthiness of women. She only intended to be the family doctor, *her* family's doctor. But this modest ambition was set aside for a larger one the night after she arrived in Whitemouth. In the absence of a qualified physician, David Ross had been acting as local doctor, both in the railway camps and now in the lumber camps, and over the years he had gained a reputation for being extremely competent. It was therefore to him that a group of workmen brought their sick companion that night in 1881.

For the first time, David didn't have to rely on his own First Aid methods. Proudly he told the men that a real doctor had come to live in Whitemouth — which cheered them considerably, until David said that she was in the next room and he would go and fetch her. *She! Her!* What to do? Get out now before any harm was done? Would Mr Ross be very offended? But the men weren't quick enough. Before they had made up their minds, 'Mrs Doctor' had walked briskly into the room, examined the sick man and prescribed his cure.

This first patient followed Mrs Doctor's advice and he duly recovered, but his recovery was not accompanied by the instant conversion of the entire neighbourhood. It took time. But, little by little, the sick and injured increasingly called at the Ross cabin for her ministrations, rather than his, and gradually news of Charlotte's medical work spread to all the camps in the area. And beyond. In spite of their own medicine men, some of the Indians would bring their sick as much as forty miles by canoe for a consultation with Dr Ross.

At first most of her patients were men, a unique situation. Charlotte was probably the only woman doctor in Canada at this time whose practice was composed largely of males. And she was one of the few doctors who had to cope with injuries more often than diseases. Most of the people who called on her services were victims of logging accidents and they were brought to her with deep axe-wounds in their feet or legs. But occasionally the wounds were in other places — and from other causes.

As soon as the lumbermen moved into an area, the publicans also moved in, and during Charlotte's first years at Whitemouth she had to deal with injuries from slogging incidents as well as from logging accidents. In the evenings the men would often get fighting drunk, and in fact David considered them so dangerous that he insisted Charlotte keep the door bolted whenever he was away from home. After the land had been cleared, when most of the lumbermen had moved on and settler families had moved in, this was no longer necessary, but during those first years a woman wasn't safe, even such a respected woman as Mr Ross's wife. She certainly wouldn't go out alone after dark, and she wisely refused to do so the night what sounded like a whole saloonful of drunks came banging on her door, calling for the doctor. David wasn't home, Charlotte didn't know any of the men, and she didn't trust them. If this was a real emergency, they could fetch someone she did know, someone she could rely on. Only then would she answer the saloon call.

In fact it was a genuine emergency. A suitably sober ex-patient was sent for to vouch for this and to chaperone the lady doctor to the scene of the bloodshed, so Mrs Dr Ross allowed herself to be hurried out of the cabin and down to the saloon. There she found a man bleeding profusely from a deep wound in his neck. He was apparently anaesthetized by the drink he had taken, for he sat calmly in a chair and even offered helpful suggestions while Dr Ross sewed up the wound with an ordinary needle and thread — the only suitable instruments she had with her. While she was doing so, the more sober customers took turns in holding the lantern — but one by one they either fainted or retired to be sick. This sewing bee was too much for them. The man's neck was tough as leather from years of exposure to the climate and Dr Ross was having to use all her strength to get the needle through the skin. A gruesome scene and enough to cause the most stalwart to faint. But on went the lady doctor, clenching her teeth, digging in the needle — and when, finally, the job was done and she was washing the needle and tucking it back into her case, there was another incident. The police arrived and arrested her patient for brawling.

The patient was escorted away, but he never forgot how Dr Ross had come to his aid with a stitch in time, and neither did those who had witnessed her behaviour. Each case she dealt with so nervelessly and so pluckily increased her reputation and gradually even the most sceptical of the he-men were boasting proudly of David Ross's courageous and unusual wife who would brave all weathers, just like a man, to sew up a wound or treat a diphtheria case or deliver a baby.

Dr Ross delivered a great many babies as her practice grew, for she worked in Whitemouth for more than thirty years and during that time it developed into a stable and sober community of homesteader families. But although it might be stable, Whitemouth was still only in the first stage of settlement. There were few roads that could be called roads. Sometimes Dr Ross had to visit her patients by canoe; at other times it was by ox team or by horse, and in winter she travelled by sleigh. It was a great luxury when a patient lived along the railway line and Dr Ross could actually make her call by train.

During these years, Charlotte Ross had as many male as female patients, but she remained very much a woman doctor. That is, she did all the womanly things as well as the medical ones. Often, when she went to deliver a child, she would stay on for a few hours, scrub the floors, do the laundry and cook enough food to last the family for a day or two, before making her journey home from the isolated homestead she had been visiting. She dealt with the total emergency, not merely with the medical one, and if she could help her patient by doing the housework, then she did the housework. Naturally this was greatly appreciated, and it was accepted with far less surprise than other examples of her femininity. How could she discuss cooking recipes with a farmer's wife while scrubbing up after amputating the husband's leg? It was incongruously domestic. So was her love of embroidery and knitting. The type of woman who would dig a pathway through the snow in sub-zero weather wasn't expected to be wearing hand-embroidered petticoats while she did so, petticoats which she had stitched herself.

Charlotte's clothes were far more fashionable than those of her neighbours and many of them were ordered from Montreal. But they were always functional. Generally she wore a black skirt and a white blouse, so that with a quick change of blouse she would be crisp and ready to set off anywhere at a moment's notice. All the same, it did seem odd that after returning from a call she would spend the evening knitting, or would stay up half the night so that she could thump down the bread and see it safely in and out of the bread oven.

It seemed odd, but it met with approval. One of the reasons for Charlotte's popularity in the district was that she was such a womanly woman. She didn't offend the conventions. She might exhibit as much bravery and initiative as any man, but at heart she was a wife and mother, and that's what women were expected to be at Whitemouth. She scrubbed and polished and baked and sewed just as a wife should, and she made a secure and happy home for her family in that log cabin on the river bank. Maybe you could see the stars through the roof in the summer and watch the snow sift through in the winter, but inside everything was warm and cosy. And outside there was a garden full of roses — the first ever grown in Manitoba.

David Ross built a frame house for his family in 1898 and this wasn't only because of the cracks in the roof — his children were growing both in size and number. Charlotte adored children and she had eight in all, but one of the boys died while she was still at Whitemouth. It was while he was dying that she made what must have been one of the most courageous decisions of her life. She was at his bedside, knowing that his death was imminent, when she was called urgently to a confinement case. Dr Ross had every excuse for refusing to answer the call. Her own small son needed her, she was seven months pregnant, and in addition the snow was so thick outside that it was almost impassable. But out she went to see someone whom she could help. On the way the snow was so deep that the men had to halt the sleigh and shovel a path for the horses — and this amazing woman shovelled away with them. Fortunately she reached her patient in time, and also returned home in time, just a few hours before her little boy died.

Dr Ross gave birth to one final child, long after the others, when she was nearly fifty — a girl who was also named Charlotte. This child was the same age as Dr Ross's granddaughter, Edith, who was also to become a doctor. None of Dr Ross's own children became doctors. Perhaps they had seen too much of what it entailed.

The interesting thing about Charlotte Ross is that although she was a most dedicated doctor, she had never intended to be a general practitioner. She merely wanted to be qualified to treat her own family. And, in a way, this is what she was doing all those years: ministering to an extended family which just happened to have spread itself across a hundred miles or so of territory. Her husband had a similar sense of responsibility to the whole neighbourhood, rather than to his immediate household only. While Charlotte was busy doctoring, he was busy providing Whitemouth with a school-house and churches. David was a sterner character than Charlotte but, like her, he was a devout Presbyterian and one of the first buildings he provided at Whitemouth was a small cabin which was to act as church and Sunday school, as well as community centre and school. Visiting theological students took the services and Charlotte ran the Sunday school.

She continued to run the Sunday school until she left White-mouth in 1912. And it was only then, after her husband had died, that she gave up her medical practice. She was nearly seventy by this time, old enough to retire even by the standards of pioneering women doctors. She moved to Winnipeg[12] where many of her children and grandchildren were living.

If Charlotte had been younger when her husband died, she might have set up a practice in Winnipeg. She was qualified to do so. She was licensed in Manitoba and although it was an unusual licence it was valid. As Whitemouth was near the border between the provinces of Manitoba and Ontario, and as there had been some doubt as to which province would eventually claim the settlement, Charlotte had applied to the Manitoba Legislature for permission to practise medicine. Legally, she was therefore well qualified to establish an office in Winnipeg.

But Winnipeg didn't need physicians as desperately as White-mouth had done; the city didn't even lack women doctors. It could

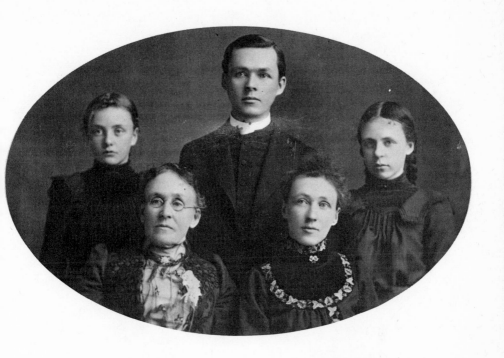

Front row (left to right): Dr Charlotte Ross with her daughter Minnie. Back row: Dr Ross's youngest daughter Lottie, Minnie's husband Hope and their daughter, the future Dr Edith Ross

Dr Amelia Yeomans

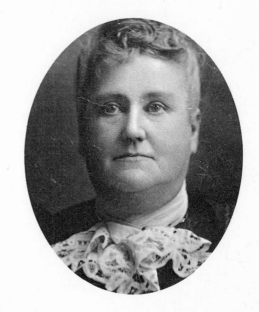

have done with more, but they were no novelty. Back in the 1880's the two stalwarts, Amelia and Lilian Yeomans had led the way as Winnipeg's first women physicians. Both had made an impression on the city, as much by their suffrage and temperance campaigning as by their medical work. They were very different characters from home-loving Charlotte Ross.

Why the Yeomans ladies should have decided to take up medicine is easy to understand. Amelia's husband — Lilian's father — had been an army surgeon in the American Civil War and it was after his death that the two women went off to Ann Arbor in Michigan to study for their degree.[13] Lilian enrolled at Ann Arbor in 1879, a year before Amelia,[14] and this produced an unusual sequence of events: the daughter graduated first, and thus predated her mother.

Lilian received her MD degree in 1882 and was registered with Manitoba's College of Physicians and Surgeons (by examination) on September 20 of the same year.[15] She lost no time in getting to work. Only two days later, on September 22, she was announcing in the *Winnipeg Free Press* that she had opened a practice in Midwifery and Diseases of Women and Children.[16] Amelia wasn't so quick off the mark. Although she graduated the following year and although she seems to have begun her practice almost immediately, it wasn't until 1885 that she received her licence.

The delay in getting registered may well have been because Amelia refused to sit the exam. As a stalwart suffragette, she would have found the oral almost as unpalatable as Emily Stowe had done. However, she did eventually take the exam — she wasn't quite as anti-male as Dr Stowe. The motto of the suffrage club which Amelia Yeomans founded in Manitoba was 'Peace on earth, good will towards men,'[17] and it was no accident that she chose this text. She did show good will towards men.

On one occasion, she gave a public lecture to men only, an unlikely thing for a suffragette to do. But it soon became very obvious why women had been excluded from the gathering. Dr Yeomans' topic was the depravity of Winnipeg, and she spoke with a characteristic, but un-Victorian frankness, describing a recent visit to one of the city's hospitals, where she had seen 'young girls made to suffer through the wickedness of men, their young lives ruined, while their betrayers moved untarnished in any rank of society.' Reading between the lines of the carefully phrased newspaper re-

port about this lecture,[18] it sounds as if Dr Yeomans went into
considerable detail about the effects of venereal disease. Not a
delicate subject for ladies to listen to.

The lecture was given to a large audience at Selkirk Hall, and it
was well received. For Dr Amelia was an extremely clever woman.
She didn't berate the men for their licentious behaviour. She ap-
pealed to their chivalry and begged them to protect innocent young
maidens as they would their own daughters. Many of the audience
left the hall praising the doctor's frankness, and fired with the determination to be Sir Galahad to any stray maiden who didn't even
look as if she might be in distress.

Amelia Yeomans' frankness was not appreciated so wholeheartedly when she turned her attentions to a female audience, publish-
ing a pamphlet, through the Woman's Christian Temperance
Union (WCTU), specifically warning young ladies about the 'pitfalls'
of city life. This pamphlet was considered indecently outspoken.
How could a lady doctor write such a tract? And how could the
WCTU sponsor it? It was both offensive and disgusting. Dr Yeomans
found herself under attack in her own camp until Father Drum-
mond, a fellow reformer, publicly supported the leaflet, insisting
that 'fear of consequences was one of the most powerful deterrents
the world knew.'[19]

Amelia Yeomans is said to have been the first person to campaign
against the 'white slave traffic' in Winnipeg, and this was certainly
one of her main Causes. Apart from medicine, she had three principal causes: female suffrage, the Woman's Christian Temperance
Union and the fight against prostitution — and naturally all three
were related. Women couldn't hope to attain equality while their
husbands were coming home roaring drunk and spending their
wages on alcohol instead of on the education of their children. Nor
would women ever be respected as equals while they were allowing
their bodies — the Human Form Divine — to serve the baser in-
stincts of exploitive males. Reform was therefore needed in all
areas, and particularly in the home. Dr. Yeomans believed very
strongly in the beneficial influence of the home — the orderly,
Christian, teetotal home. If men spent more time at home, she said,
they would be more fitted to remedy the social evils of their national
home. But as things stood at present, it was women who were most
suited to govern the nation, because women were at home more

and therefore had a more godly and philanthropic approach to life.
Strong words for the 1890's.

But Dr Yeomans was very much a woman of her time. Born in Quebec, in 1842, she had been brought up in the Canadas and had come west with the wave of reformers who moved across the Prairies in the wake of the railway builders, trying to establish some order and decency. There was plenty for her to do in Winnipeg, and not only as a doctor. Towards the end of the nineteenth century, Winnipeg was known as one of the wickedest cities in Canada,[20] and it was also becoming one of the largest. Between 1881 and 1901, the population of the city increased from about eight thousand to more than forty-two thousand. Everyone travelling west passed through Winnipeg, and many stayed, for there was so much building going on that any healthy man could find work there, without having to brave the discomforts of frontier life in the unsettled land farther west.

Most of the new citizens were male, young and lusty single males or young and lusty grass-widowers who wanted to play hard as well as working hard. As their numbers grew, so did the numbers of bars and brothels. When Dr Yeomans was campaigning in Winnipeg there was a saloon on just about every corner, and McFarlane Street and Annabella Street were notorious for their many Houses of Ill Fame. However, it is doubtful if there was as much 'white slaving' as Dr Yeomans imagined. Most of the prostitutes seem to have chosen their profession, rather than being lured into it. But all the more reason to lead them into righteous paths. And into paths which would be less of a health hazard.

Dr Yeomans and her fellow reformers had sporadic success. Prohibition wasn't legislated until 1916, after she had died, but at least she managed to get some measures taken to restrict prostitution. Until the reformers became active the police had been turning a blind eye, or at least a myopic eye, accepting both prostitution and drunkenness as inevitable facts of life. What else could you expect when there were so many healthy young men around? 'Temperance,' replied the reformers, 'virtue and sobriety.' The reformers grew in strength and numbers in the 1890's and 1900's and they began to attract so much public support that gradually the police were forced to act, to make arrests more often and to impose more than token fines. The days of Winnipeg's wickedness were waning.

Dr Yeomans was one of the most active members of this reform movement. She enlisted the support of the city fathers, pressured the police, wrote to the newspapers and was always ready to speak to any group that could be gathered to hear her. She was apparently a very witty speaker, making her points clearly and often amusingly — you didn't fall asleep when Amelia Yeomans was giving a lecture. And you weren't allowed to sleep afterwards either. Dr Amelia's speeches were given to stir you into action, and she saw to it that there was action. Whatever the cause, she was a tireless agitator. When she died, in 1913, E. Cora Hind wrote: 'There should be a lifesized portrait of Dr Amelia Yeomans placed in the city hall, for it is very questionable if any worshipful mayor whose portrait now adorns the walls ever did one tithe as much for the real up-building of the city.'[21]

This is an overstatement — as it was bound to be, considering the author — but it is not so far from the truth. Amelia Yeomans did 'up-build' the city in a great many areas. Like the Stowes, she would fight against any injustice, and champion any cause that aroused her sense of rightness. The poor and underprivileged, men as well as women, all found a friend in Amelia Yeomans, and it says as much for her character as for her Christianity that a condemned man in Winnipeg jail asked to have Amelia, rather than a priest, as his spiritual adviser.[22]

Winnipeg's Icelandic community also looked to her when they were in need. Around the turn of the century, there were more Icelanders in Winnipeg than any other group of foreign-born immigrants, and Dr Yeomans was particularly interested in their problems. In Iceland, women had the vote. When they settled in Canada, they had to relinquish this privilege. Here was a ready-made cause. But Dr Yeomans did more than campaign for their suffrage. She was one of the earliest people to draw attention to the problems of the non-English-speakers who settled in Canada.

In all these causes, Amelia was supported by her daughter Dr Lilian Yeomans, but — like her sisters — Lilian lived in the shadow of her mother. Lilian may have been the first to practise in Winnipeg, but when people spoke of Dr Yeomans, they meant Amelia. An obituary notice in the *Calgary Herald*[23] doesn't even credit Lilian with being a physician. It speaks of her as 'Miss Lilian Yeomans of the post office inspector's department.'

However, this may have been because neither Lilian nor her mother registered themselves as physicians when they moved to Calgary. They had retired from medicine when they settled there. Amelia moved to Calgary in 1905 and Lilian followed a couple of years later,[24] and neither of them went there as campaigners in medicine. But they did go there as campaigners: there was plenty of suffrage and temperance work to be done in Calgary. When Amelia died at the age of seventy-one, she was still serving these two causes. She was Vice-President of the Dominion wctu, honorary Vice-President of the Ottawa Equal Suffrage Society and honorary President of the Calgary Suffrage Association.

Amelia may well have felt that her work for women in medicine had already been done. Certainly there was not the opposition that there used to be. Two young ladies had recently opened a practice in Calgary without any apparent difficulty and, even more significant, these two young ladies had graduated in Canada. It did look as if the most important battle had been won, the battle for the medical education of women. By 1913, when Amelia Yeomans died, more than two hundred women had already graduated in medicine *in Canada*.

This is an imposing figure, but it doesn't follow that there was a woman doctor in almost every town. Female medical graduates might no longer be a novelty, but female doctors were still rather rare. This was because many of our women found work in the United States — there was so much more opportunity there. Others married and never practised medicine. But by far the largest group of expatriate practitioners were the missionaries. By 1913 at least a quarter of all the women who had studied medicine in Canada had done so expressly so that they could serve usefully in the mission field. Within a year of their graduation they had set off for India or China, or some distant part of the world where their lives could be guaranteed to be far tougher and more insecure than that of even the most hardy pioneers.

The missionary journals of the period make dauntless reading. Discomfort and death haunt the pages. Here's young Lucinda Graham arriving in Shanghai in 1891,[25] only a few months after receiving her md cm (Trinity). She treks inland to Honan, spurred on by a crusading zeal to Conquer China for Christ, but she can't begin to do so until she has mastered the language — and she is still translating from the Chinese when she herself is 'translated to higher service'. This second translation was due to a virulent type of cholera which killed her within twenty-four hours, and which threatened the lives of all too many missionaries. Others were to die from plague or typhus — or just plain murder.

Yet the journals are not so much depressing as overpowering. Even when describing the most ghastly experiences, they tell such a story of triumph that, at the end, when they recount how 'all the trumpets sounded on the other side' to greet these valiant women, one can't help wishing one had a trumpet too, so that one could join in the fanfare and applaud, from this side, such unquestioning and unquestionable heroism.

MEDICAL MARITIMERS

ANNIE ISABELLE HAMILTON (Dalhousie, 1894)

Dalhousie's first woman medical graduate, Annie Hamilton, has been described as a 'fiery, determined little individual.' As a student, she tried to convert her male classmates to feminism and teetotalism (without any success at all) and after her graduation she used to ride a bicycle, wearing a divided skirt, when she made her house calls. This drew attention to her causes as well as to herself. She practised in Halifax, among the poor of the city, until 1903 when she left Canada to become a medical missionary in China. Halifax was sad. Annie had been a popular eccentric.

JANE HEARTZ BELL (New York, 1893)

Dr Jane Heartz (Mrs Bell) graduated from the Woman's Medical College of the New York Infirmary for Women and Children in 1893 and then took postgraduate work at Johns Hopkins University. Returning to Canada, she took over Dr Angwin's practice in Halifax. She was an active social worker and, in addition to running a practice for women and children, she held senior appointments on the Welfare Council, the YWCA, the Community Chest, the Children's Aid Society, the Protestant Orphanage and the Maritimes School of Social Work. In 1950 Dalhousie awarded her an honorary LL D. She died in 1963 at the age of 94.

VICTORIA ERNST (Dalhousie, 1900)

When Victoria Ernst was at Dalhousie, she was known by the students as 'Victoria, by the Grace of God, Miss Ernst' (she seemed as old as the Queen; she was 44 when she graduated, having taught school at Bridgewater for many years). Dr Ernst ran a general practice in Halifax and, although she didn't marry, she adopted several boys, choosing the most difficult and unwanted boys in the orphanage. When she retired from medicine, she took up real estate, proving so successful at it that, when she died in 1940, she was said to be the largest taxpayer in the city.

GRACE RICE (Dalhousie, 1903)

Grace Rice took postgraduate work in Dublin after her graduation (specializing in obstetrics and gynaecology) and returned to Halifax in 1911. She became well known throughout the Maritimes for her work in paediatrics as well as in obstetrics and gynaecology. She died at her home in Halifax in 1963.

MINNA MAY AUSTEN (Dalhousie, 1903)
Dr Austen was one of Dalhousie's early missionaries, serving at Chengtu in
West China with the Methodist mission there. She became seriously ill in
China and was obliged to return home after ten years. In spite of her ill health
she began to work again at the time of the Halifax Explosion, when every
available doctor was needed, but the pressure was too much for her and she
became very ill. She died in 1923 at the age of 45.

ANNIE HENNIGAR SANFORD (Dalhousie, 1906)
Annie Hennigar (Mrs Sanford) was an artist as well as a physician. She was
born at Noel, N.S., in 1873 and she died there in 1950. She was a horse-and-
buggy doctor, travelling in all weather and across rough country to cope
with every type of emergency, acting as surgeon, physician, dentist (she was
known as 'a grand man with a tooth'). On one occasion she had to blindfold
her horses with her carriage rug to get them to pass two bears on a lonely road.

JEMIMA MACKENZIE (Dalhousie, 1904) and MARY MACKENZIE SMITH
(Dalhousie, 1905)
These two sisters both became missionaries in India and Jemima was awarded
the Kaisar-i-Hind and an LLD from Dalhousie. Mary retired from missionary
work when she married in 1911. She settled in Ontario, where she worked as
medical inspector of public schools.

6

Healing for Christ

IN THE late nineteenth century, there were two main fields that
attracted Canadian missionaries: India and China. Africa wasn't
really on the books yet, since most of that continent was only just
being 'opened up' — and those areas which had already been opened
were well controlled by the London Missionary Society. There
were, of course, other heathen lands which required missionaries,
and a few of our women doctors went to such places as Honolulu or
Korea, but for the most part they went to China or India because
that was where Canada had established its overseas missions. Many
of the missions were medical, and this was not only because trained
physicians were greatly needed in the east. It was also because healing drew attention and attracted converts. If you brought sight to
the blind by removing cataracts, the gospel message began to have
a very real impact.

Where any doctor was sent depended largely on which missionary society sent her and to which church she belonged, for heathen
lands had been divided into national and denominational spheres
of interest. For instance, if you went to India with the American
Union Women's Missionary Society, as two of our Nova Scotian
doctors did, then you might find yourself working at Fatepur in
the north. If you went with the Anglicans, like the Toronto graduate Mildred Jean Haslam, then you could be stationed farther
north, at Kangra. Elizabeth Beatty was sent to Indore, because the
Canadian Presbyterians had conversion rights to that area. And

several women doctors worked along the east coast of Central India, because that was Canadian Baptist territory.

It was all carefully worked out to avoid overlapping and to spread the net as widely as possible, but the Roman Catholics don't seem to have been in on the plan. Sometimes they established rival missions in Occupied Territory, drawing converts away from the Protestants by offering better soup or more careful instruction. In China it was more often the Protestants who were the interlopers, and when a Canadian mission moved into an area known as Unoccupied Territory, it might well find a group of Catholic sisters already established there. All became sisters, fellow sufferers, during the various outbreaks of anti-foreign riots, but in the more peaceable interludes it was fair game to reconvert Christians by offering superior medical or educational facilities — even if one was aware that a depressing number of converts were influenced by material rather than spiritual motives.

The more accessible parts of the Chinese Empire were therefore well infiltrated by the end of the nineteenth century, but there were still a few areas on its outer perimeter which were entirely Unoccupied. One of these was the mountainous land of Tibet. A French Lazarist, the Abbé Huc, had journeyed through Tibet between 1844 and 1846, and, in 1892, Annie Taylor, an evangelizing English Protestant, had braved its fearsome mountains in order to bring the gospel to the Tibetans.[1] But neither had established a permanent mission. Millions of Tibetans had never heard the gospel message, had never even heard the name of Christ. Here was a challenging, wide-open field for anyone who cared or dared to take it on.

It was a young Canadian woman who took up the challenge. She was Susanna Carson Rijnhart, daughter of J.S. Carson of Strathroy and wife of the Dutch missionary, Petrus Rijnhart.[2] Susie Carson seems to have known, very early in life, that it was her vocation to be a medical missionary. She was an eager young Methodist, very active in the Epworth League in Strathroy and London, and when she was only fourteen she had already decided on medical training — her father had been one of the eleven people who had answered Elizabeth Smith's advertisement in 1879.[3] Mr Carson had been extremely interested to hear of the projected medical course at Queen's and he wrote to Miss Smith that he was 'heartily in sympathy' with it — but his daughter would not be able to take part in its first session. She was far too young, he said. She hadn't finished her schooling yet; she still had to pass her intermediate *and* take up the study of the Classics. So, perhaps later . . . .

Later, when Susie was old enough to go to college, the Woman's Medical College had been opened in Toronto, and she enrolled there, probably because it was nearer. She was one of its earliest students, graduating in 1888, in the second class of women ever to do so from the Toronto college.[4] Six years later, when she was still in her twenties — she was no hardened veteran — she married Petrus Rijnhart, said farewell to her family and set off with her husband for unoccupied, unconquered and unpenetrated Tibet.

Tibet was not only unpenetrated: it was virtually impenetrable. Although the Abbé Huc and Miss Taylor had managed to gain entry to the interior, very few Europeans of any type had ever visited the country. Fewer still had survived a visit. For Tibet was a closed land, sealed off from the West by its mountains and by its suspicion of foreigners. Europeans were simply not admitted. The border with India was closely guarded against any expansion by the British, so entry from there was out of the question — you would be recognized as an invader before you had found your way through the first mountain pass.

However, it was possible to slip in unobserved if you came through China. There was less vigilance on that border, for Tibet was a form of vassal state of the Chinese Empire. Both the Abbé Huc and Annie Taylor had used the Chinese route, and in fact Petrus Rijnhart had already done so too. He had made an exploratory journey into eastern Tibet in 1892, and he had met no opposition. Nor had he been stopped in China. There was a strong European presence there, and although the Chinese hated 'foreign devils', they were powerless to keep them out.

Susie and Petrus therefore decided to enter Tibet through China,[5] even though they would have to travel the full breadth of the Empire before crossing into Tibet. That was quite an ordeal in itself. They did the first part of their journey up the Yangtse, by British steamer, but when they left the Yangtse they were less protected and far less comfortable. First they travelled by houseboat, then overland by cart, and finally by horse and donkey. They wore Chinese dress in order to attract the minimum of attention — a ruse that failed in its purpose when Susie first donned her disguise. She mistook one of the undergarments for an overgarment and attracted far more notice than if she had worn western clothes. Fortunately this shocking display of lingerie took place when the couple were still a long way from Tibet.

The Rijnharts were accompanied on their journey by a fellow missionary, William Ferguson, but although he entered Tibet with them and helped them set up the mission, he returned to China after a few months. This was more significant than it seemed at the time: if Mr Ferguson had stayed, the final tragedy of the Rijnhart's mission might have been avoided. Murder and misery were to result from their venture into unoccupied territory.

As first-line missionaries in such a hostile part of the world as Tibet, both Susie and Petrus were prepared to die for their Faith, but it is doubtful if either of them really expected to do so. When they crossed into Tibet in 1895, they had joy in their hearts — and firearms for protection. They weren't seeking martyrdom. They had come to this heathen land to offer a long life of service, and they had brought a lifetime's supplies with them: cooking utensils, clothing, dental and surgical instruments, medicines and drugs, photographic equipment, copies of the Scriptures in Tibetan, and even a sewing machine and a bicycle. They had provided most of these goods themselves, for they had not been sent by any of the missionary societies. Tibet was to remain an Unoccupied Field.

Susie and Petrus would have found this hard to believe during the first years of their mission, for they were well received by the Tibetans and were allowed to build a house in the very heart of the lama country, about twenty miles inside the border at a small village called Lusar. Lusar was, in effect, the shopping centre for the great lamasery of Kumbum, which was one of the great centres of Buddhist learning, one of the holiest and most famous monasteries in all of Asia.

Besides being holy, Kumbum was also very beautiful. It was set in a fertile valley and the square houses of the lamas climbed the slopes of the hills on either side. There were more than four thousand lamas living at Kumbum and each had his own house, which he kept shining white by climbing onto the roof and pouring buckets of whitewash over it. As the buildings rose up the hill, terrace upon terrace, they increased in size and splendour, the larger dwellings at the top being coloured red rather than white. And the most important building of all was 'a thousand brilliant colours'. This was the golden-roofed temple, one of the most splendid and holy temples in the entire Buddhist world. It contained a huge Buddha which was said to be made of solid gold, and it had all the trappings: hundreds of butter lamps, almost as many prayer wheels, and thousands upon thousands of worshippers who had come from as far away as Peking to kowtow before the Great Buddha.

Since so many pilgrims came to worship at Kumbum, it also attracted merchants, and the secular town of Lusar had become one of the main trading centres in Tibet. North met south here, and east met west. It was a major crossroads. The Rijnharts could hardly have found a more strategic location for their mission.

Their house in Lusar was only about five minutes' walk from the Kumbum lamasery, and it is surprising that they managed to establish themselves so near to such an important religious centre — for they were, of course, recognized as foreigners. But they seem to have been regarded as friendly visitors rather than as foreign devils. They began their medical work immediately, and this gave them a favourable reputation, but more important was that they conducted their missionary work with great tact. Both Susie and Petrus were very likeable people, far more tolerant than the average nineteenth-century missionary, and it wasn't their policy to desecrate shrines or break idols. They felt that all religions deserved respect, even the most misguided, and they were prepared to recognize Buddhism as a religion and even admire some of its ceremonies.

They thoroughly enjoyed the Butter God Festival, the occasion when a twenty-foot image of Buddha — made of solid butter — was on display in the temple. Maybe they found it symbolic when the heat from the many lamps gradually melted the effigy, but they didn't try to prevent the Tibetans celebrating the occasion. Nor did they rail against other traditional ceremonies. In fact, they found some extremely impressive, especially the 'nocturnal devotions' when the entire population of Kumbum and Lusar would go up onto their rooftops and pray all night. These devotions were both colourful and aromatic, fragrant with incense and lit by thousands of red paper lanterns. They were also extremely noisy. Opening with loud blasts on a horn and punctuated by the sound of gongs, cymbals and bells, the devotions would go on all night, while the whole valley resounded with the chanting of prayers, the singing of hymns, the click of prayer wheels and the telling of rosaries. With four thousand lamas and as many laiety all on their rooftops worshipping so loudly and energetically, sleep for the Rijnharts would be impossible. Yet they were impressed by the sincerity of the worshippers. How could one object, when so many were praying so fervently?

Susie even admired the golden-tiled temple. She was permitted to enter it on the one day of the year when women were allowed in — a unique privilege for a non-Buddhist, and a foreigner at that. Her reaction was very typical. She was fascinated by the pilgrims, impressed by their faith and saddened by the misdirection of their devotion.

'There is something pathetic in this spectacle of heathen worship,' she wrote, 'and it is not, in my opinion, the part of the Christian missionary to assume an air of ridicule and contempt for the religious ideas and practices of peoples less enlightened than his own; for in every religious service, however absurd or degraded from the Christian view-point, there is some feeble acknowledgement and groping after the one great God.'[6]

This, of course, was why the Rijnharts didn't launch a frontal attack on Buddhism. They recognized it as a sincere religion, so it deserved to be treated with respect. But, in any case, it wasn't in their nature to condemn or to hate. Many missionaries would have felt impelled to destroy the great image of Buddha, but Susie and Petrus took a more subtle approach, decorating the walls of their waiting room and surgery with Bible pictures — illustrations of the Good Samaritan or of Lazarus being risen from the dead — so that the Tibetans would ask for explanations, ask to hear the gospel stories and be weaned rather than forced from their heathen ways. This policy proved very successful. Word began to get around that these friendly foreign healers had a form of religious knowledge that had somehow escaped the Tibetans, and a great many of the lamas became curious to hear more.

The most curious was the *kanpo*, the abbot of the lamasery, a young man called Mina Fuyeh. He was a 'living Buddha', the greatest dignitary in all of northeastern Tibet, and before long he was actually inviting the Rijnharts to his residence. Susie and Petrus had been learning Tibetan from a very junior lama, a youth called Ishinima, and he accused them of lying when he heard of the invitation. It was impossible, he said. No foreigners would ever be admitted to such a holy place. It was an unheard of privilege.

Maybe, but the Rijnharts were expected there in a few hours. The pretext for their visit was to cure the abbot's treasurer, but after they had treated the treasurer, Susie and Petrus were ushered into Mina Fuyeh's presence and were shown very great courtesy. He remained on his throne — that was only fitting — but he seated his visitors on two beautiful rugs, offered them tea in delicate china basins, and put himself out to be agreeable. Needless to say, the missionaries were on their best behaviour and they politely stirred rancid butter into their tea, a custom they found most unpalatable, while they chatted with the abbot.

It seems to have been a chat more than a formal discourse, for Mina Fuyeh was a lively young man. Although he had accumulated a great many years as well as considerable sanctity in his previous lives, he had only lived twenty-seven years of his present life so he was much the same age as the missionaries. And he had a common interest with them: religion. It was a highly successful visit and it was to be the first of many others. This was the beginning of a firm friendship which developed between one sweet-natured Dutchman, one kindly Canadian girl from Strathroy . . . and the greatest dignitary in all northeastern Tibet. Soon Mina Fuyeh was dropping all formality when he was alone with the couple and, later in the same year, when the neighbouring Mohammedans rose in revolt, he invited his missionary friends to come and live in the lamasery, offering them two large rooms and a kitchen in his own residence. They would be safe with him, he said, even if Lusar was attacked.

From then on Susie and Petrus could do no wrong. They were wards of the abbot, so no harm could come to them, not from the locals at any rate. But the Mohammedans had started what threatened to be a full-scale war, pillaging towns, slaughtering every Infidel in their path and even threatening the safety of the monastery at Kumbum. At that time there were about ten million Moslems in the Chinese Empire and many of them lived inside Tibet. As a minority group, they had well-found grudges — they were barely tolerated by the Buddhists — and the slightest incident could flare into revolt.

The present revolt looked very serious. The whole countryside was in turmoil and the refugees flocked into Kumbum for protection. The Chinese sent an army to head off the Moslem forces, and the lamas put aside their priestly robes and rode out in a body to add their strength to the Chinese force. Their departure from Kumbum was a splendid affair and most of the neighbourhood gathered on the rooftops to cheer them off to war. The lamas were dressed in red and yellow, with red silk turbans on their heads, and shining swords (and even guns) in their hands. An imposing sight. And they were accompanied by the usual noise, the beating of gongs and drums, the click of prayer wheels and the incantation of the Buddhist prayer *om mani padme hum*. As they set off so bravely to battle, some Christian prayers were also offered for their safety: the two 'white lamas' were up on a rooftop among the throng, wishing 'God speed' to the troops.

The two white lamas, as they had come to be called, were very busy at this time, for the increased population brought them an almost impossible number of patients. A serious diphtheria epidemic broke out in Kumbum, the result of so many people crowding into the monastery, and there were also hundreds of wounded to be treated. This was a grizzly business. Some of the refugees were barely alive when they staggered into Kumbum (one young lad had sixteen spear wounds in his side) and they told terrible stories of atrocities, of women being raped, villages burned and babies stuck with spears. Susie shivered with horror as she heard these tales and thanked the Lord that she had been given sanctuary at Kumbum. Before long, however, she and her husband were to be called out to the battlefield. The Buddhists had won the day, but they had suffered heavy casualties.

Susie and Petrus didn't relish the idea of riding to within a mile of the Mohammedan lines, but apparently they 'hesitated not'. They thought of the suffering of 'our lama soldiers' (they had fully identified with the lamas), they remembered how our lama soldiers had risked their lives to defend helpless women and children, and they also remembered that they themselves were the servants of Him who went about healing all that were oppressed. So they packed up their surgical instruments and medical equipment, and rode out into the countryside, escorted by a small but heavily armed guard.

They arrived on the battlefield shortly after dawn, and for a day and a half they worked almost non-stop, amputating limbs and removing bullets. It was only around noon of the second day that they finished all the emergency treatment and then, as a reward for their labours, they were invited to a luncheon party with the Chinese general. He seems to have been rather a dubious character. Although he was a representative of the Imperial Government, he was suspected of having made a deal with the rebels, for he had unaccountably halted the fighting just when the Chinese and lama armies were in a position to deal the final blow to the opposing forces. Money was said to have changed hands. Certainly the Moslems were allowed to escape. They had slipped away in the night and reassembled — and they launched their counterattack in the middle of lunch.

Suddenly all was noise and frenzy again. The lamas seized their swords and rushed into the fray, yelling their war cry 'Sha Sha!' (eat meat!) — and the Rijnharts seized their horses and set out for home. Again they were provided with an armed guard, but it was not a large one, not nearly as large as the force of rebel horsemen that wheeled to cut them off. Susie writes that they galloped for their lives, and this was literally what they were doing. They galloped all the way back to the lamasery, pursued by the Sons of the Prophet and never knowing, when they entered a defile in the hills, if there would be another group of Moslems waiting to cut them off — and up — at the other end.

When eventually they rode exhaustedly into Kumbum, they found almost as many people gathered to welcome them as had gathered to see the great lama army off to battle a few days earlier. The people of Kumbum had heard of the counterattack and they had been waiting anxiously on their rooftops for the return of their foreign friends. One old lama was so relieved at their safe return that he could scarcely hold back his tears as he took Petrus by the hands and told him how worried they had all been.

When one hears of such spontaneous outpourings of affection, one gets great insight into the character of the Rijnharts. They must have been very exceptional people. In the year of the Moslem rising, China was being rocked by anti-foreign riots and throughout the Chinese Empire mission property was being destroyed and missionaries were being beaten up and murdered. Yet Petrus and Susie were being lovingly protected by both Tibetans and Chinese, and had even been entertained to lunch by the Chinese commander. Their popularity was so strong that six months later, after the rebellion had been put down, and when the Moslems were being victimized just about as bloodily as they had victimized the Infidel, nobody objected when Petrus went to the Mohammedans' quarter of town to treat their wounded and diseased. His behaviour was considered strange, and many considered it unpatriotic, but the Tibetans were amazed rather than offended.

This action gave Susie and Petrus the opportunity to preach the doctrine 'Love thine enemies and do good to them that hate you.' In spite of their full-time medical work, they had never lost sight of their true mission; even when they were living at the lamasery and acting both as army surgeon and public health officer, they were also running a Bible school each Wednesday and Sunday — though they were tactful enough to do this at their house in Lusar, rather than in the lamasery proper.

Their Bible school was very popular, particularly with the women and children. Susie would play her violin, Petrus would accompany her on the concertina, and the Tibetans would sing, throatily and enthusiastically, the hymns that they had been taught. The converts were mostly Tibetans, for the Chinese tended to be sceptical. They had met foreigners before and they *knew* that these white devils were always motivated by personal gain. But few Tibetans had ever met a white foreigner, and as the first of their species, Susie and Petrus certainly showed no desire for personal gain. They had exhausted themselves treating thousands of patients during the rebellion, and they had never asked for payment. Nor had they shown any disrespect towards Buddhism, as the Chinese said they would. They had done nothing offensive. And if they talked of a Heavenly Ruler that the lamas hadn't heard of, then that was most interesting and perhaps their deity should be given more attention.

Ishinima, the young lama who had taught the Rijnharts Tibetan, was so impressed by the couple that he was convinced that they alone had saved Kumbum from the rebels. They had prayed to their Heavenly Ruler for protection, and He had answered their prayers. Ishinima decided that he too would pray to Christ and, at the Rijnharts' suggestion, he put aside the small Buddha that he had aways taken to bed with him. But he remained a lama.

So did Mina Fuyeh, though he never tired of learning more about Christ's teaching. Petrus had given him a copy of the Scriptures in Tibetan and the young abbot was fascinated and soon knew them by heart. He was so interested in Christianity and he approved of so many of its precepts that, for a while, the Rijnharts thought that they were going to have the success of converting one of the greatest powers in the land. But Mina Fuyeh was indeed one of the greatest powers, temporally as well as spiritually, and he had no desire to abdicate from such a distinguished position. Nor did he see the need to do so. He could accept Christianity and incorporate it into Buddhism without renouncing the traditional faith of his country. He decided that Jesus was a reincarnation of the Great Buddha — after all, the gospels didn't specifically deny the doctrine of reincarnation.

The Rijnharts were hardly satisfied with this, but they saw it as progress rather than blasphemy. For Mina Fuyeh was so impressed by the Christian doctrines that he was actually teaching the Faith to his lamas. Theologically, there was a lot to be desired, but at least the seed was being sown very widely, even if it didn't seem to be producing very much in the way of fruit. And undoubtedly the abbot's enthusiasm helped the missionaries with their own teaching.

Susie and Petrus were so well established at Lusar, so highly honoured and in such a promising position to make thousands of converts in due course, that it is sad that they didn't stay there and consolidate their gains. But they believed that they should *spread* the gospel. They saw themselves as itinerant missionaries. When the city of Tankar invited them to come and set up a dispensary, they took this as a Sign, sadly said goodbye to their many friends, and rented a house in Tankar — for the tiny sum of thirteen dollars a year.

In fact Tankar was only about twenty-three miles from Kumbum, so they were still in touch with their friends. Mina Fuyeh often came to visit them — which, of course, ensured their security as well as giving them great prestige. When Petrus went off to Peking for a few months, leaving Susie in Tankar, the townspeople seem to have taken her on as their special care, to be guarded and protected until her husband's return. Susie could have moved into China while Petrus was away, for there were several missions within a day or two's journey on that side of the border, but she didn't feel the need.

She was among friends in Tankar and she had plenty of work to do, so she stayed on — causing great surprise to a Swedish explorer, Dr Sven Hedin, who passed through Tankar that year.

'When I reached the house indicated,' he wrote, 'a good Chinese house with an oblong courtyard, I was met by a bareheaded young lady wearing spectacles and dressed after the Chinese manner. . . . She introduced herself as Mrs Rheinhard, an American doctor of medicine. Her husband was the Dutch missionary, Mr Rheinhard, who fully a month earlier had started for Peking. . . .

'Her husband's courage in venturing to leave her behind alone among the rabble of Ten-kar truly astonished me. But there was not so much danger perhaps after all; for through her medical knowledge and skill Mrs Rheinhard had won several friends among the native population.'[7]

Petrus' courage in leaving his wife in Tankar — or, more to the point, Susie's courage in agreeing to remain there without him — was more remarkable than Dr Hedin realized, in spite of the friendship of the townsfolk. For the bespectacled young 'American' lady was pregnant at the time. Charles Carson Rijnhart was born soon after Petrus' return.

Unfortunately, the birth of young Charles didn't cause the Rijnharts to settle down. They had lived at Tankar for nearly two years when their son was born and they were feeling far too settled. When Charles was less than two months old, the family went on an 'itinerating mission', camping in tents in the wild countryside to the west, and Susie and Petrus managed to distribute so many gospels that this excursion simply whetted their appetite for further travels. Soon they were planning a long journey to the very heart of Tibet, to Lhasa, the most sacred of all the Buddhist monasteries.

Since Susie and Petrus had been made so welcome at Kumbum, it was natural that they would feel optimistic about their chances at Lhasa. But Lhasa was nearer to India, more suspicious of white foreigners, and therefore far more carefully guarded. No Europeans were allowed anywhere near that holy city. Annie Taylor, the English missionary, had tried to enter Lhasa five years earlier and she had been turned back. So had the few others who had recently tried to gain entry. Or else they had been murdered.

Susie and Petrus knew this, they knew that they were attempting the impossible, but the Lord had already opened many doors for them and, even if they couldn't get into Lhasa, they would presumably be able to establish a mission somewhere in the far interior. So they bought twelve pack horses, loaded them with tents, food, gospels and other necessities, and set off into the mountains. They only had three companions on this journey: Rahim, a longtime servant and friend, who was travelling with them so that he could return to his distant family, and two Chinese guides — who deserted as soon as the going got tough.

It wasn't long before the going did get very tough. Beyond the lamaseries, Tibet was a very wild land, inhabited by nomadic tribes of tent-dwellers and also by a great many bandits. Most of the nomads proved friendly to the missionaries, offering them food and shelter (and being rewarded with gospels and religious pamphlets), but the bandits were a constant threat. They owed allegiance to none of the recognized authorities and they murdered as casually as they plundered. Susie, Petrus, Rahim and little Charles — such a small and vulnerable party — were easy prey to any wandering band that had seen and noted their well-laden pack horses.

The whole journey sounds madness, for the elements were as hostile as the bandits. The missionaries had to struggle through driving snowstorms, trudge up mountains and ford and swim torrential ice-cold rivers. Even when they camped for the night, they were hardly snug. Bears and wolves would prowl around the tents and, as often as not, the skies would be split with terrifying electric storms and lightning would bounce from the nearby peaks and crackle around the camp.

Inevitably and implacably disaster began to strike. First, five of the pack horses were stolen, then the party began to run short of food. And then little Charles ailed, became abnormally silent, and quietly died. Miserably, the Rijnharts buried the little body of their son on a hillside, camouflaging the grave with a boulder so that neither wild robbers nor wild animals would desecrate it. And then, with heavy hearts, but still firm in their faith, they continued their journey inland.

It was shortly after this that they were halted by a group of nomads who refused to allow them to pass. They were nearing Lhasa now, only about a week's journey away from the city, and the sentries were out everywhere. The missionaries managed to outwit their guards and slip away in the night, but they were stopped again the following day. Obviously they would never get through to Lhasa. Unwillingly, they agreed to turn back, following a south-easterly route that would take them towards China. But they didn't intend to hurry back. They would spend the winter at the nearest lamasery on their road east and establish a mission there. Something would then be gained by this journey.

Susie and Petrus needed guides to lead them to the lamasery, for they didn't know the country and their friend, Rahim, was about to leave them: his route home no longer coincided with theirs. However, the tribe of nomads was glad to supply them with guides — anything to prevent these foreigners going on to Lhasa — and they also willingly replenished the couple's supply of food. But neither the food nor the guides remained for very long. Only two weeks later the party was attacked by a band of robbers, who shot most of the pack horses and wounded most of the guides (who hastily rode away, saying they would get help). Susie and Petrus were left alone in the snow, in unknown and desolate country, convinced that they would never again see their guides, knowing that the robbers were still at hand, knowing that it would be wise to move on immediately but not knowing in which direction they should walk — and having to walk, as they only had one horse left. It was a desperate situation. They loaded as many supplies as possible on the one horse, Petrus himself carried a second load of almost equal weight, and off they trudged through the thick snow.

They were at the extreme of exhaustion when eventually, in the far distance, they saw an encampment of tents. Their hopes rose. If they could only reach those tents, then they could hire horses and buy food and move on to the lamasery that was said to be somewhere in the neighbourhood. It looked as if their troubles were over. But, when they drew near, Susie and Petrus saw that a wide river separated them from the encampment. And they were far too weary to cross it.

But at least they knew that help was at hand. Petrus could swim over the following day, and in the meantime, they would spend the night on this side of the river. Optimistically they fell asleep, warmed by a renewed surge of hope and by the layer of snow which fell on the waterproof under which they slept.

It is doubtful if Petrus ever swam that river. The following morning he waded in, but then apparently he saw some people not far away on his own side of the bank. He shouted something to Susie, which she didn't catch, he waved to her cheerfully, he shouted 'ta-ta!' and then he walked along the bank, round some rocks — and out of her life. She never saw him again.

Later, Susie decided that the people Petrus had seen were probably the robbers of the previous day and that when they saw him approaching, they thought he was out for vengeance — and killed him. It seemed the most likely explanation. But at the time, Susie wasn't worried. She wasn't even worried when Petrus didn't return that night: he had said that bargaining for horses might take some time and that he mightn't be back before dark. He had purposely left her his big revolver, just in case she had to spend the night without him. So although Susie was alone in the snow and in a very desolate part of the country, she passed the day quite cheerfully, watching a group of bears gambolling not far away and thinking happily of the mission that she and Petrus were going to establish.

But the following day she did begin to worry — searching along the river bank and scanning the hills with her telescope to see if there was any sign of Petrus. By the third day she was getting desperate. She tried to swim the river to discover if her husband had crossed to the encampment, but the current was too strong for her. Even her horse wouldn't attempt the crossing. She tried to attract the attention of the people across the river, and eventually she succeeded in doing so, but she couldn't hear what they were shouting back. But at least she had made contact with them and, the following day, they sent a man with a yak across the river so that she could ride across on the yak, using it as a sort of half-submerged boat. All her life, Susie had been terrified of cattle, an unlikely fear in such a brave woman, and climbing onto that animal and sitting on it while it swam the river was, strangely, one of the most courageous actions of her life. But it was the courage of desperation. She *had* to get news of Petrus.

She didn't manage to. When she arrived on the other side of the river, dripping, shaking, and not so very far from starving, the Tibetans could tell her nothing of Petrus. Nor were they at all welcoming at first. They weren't pleased to discover that she was a woman, and a white one at that, and they were even less pleased when they found she was enquiring about a husband who had probably been murdered. They feared they might be blamed for the deed or that their friends might be blamed. A friend might even have been responsible for the murder. At all events they weren't going to help hunt for the culprit. But they did take Susie in, and they seem to have treated her kindly, letting her stay with them almost a week while she watched the other bank with her telescope. And when it became obvious that Petrus was never going to return, they even crossed the river to fetch her supplies and then provided her with guides to take her on the first stage of her journey back to China.

Susie's return journey took her two months — on yak, horse and foot. It was a nightmare ordeal, largely because she was a woman travelling alone. She had a 'passport' which ensured that she would be provided with lodging, mounts and guides from town to town, but she was very much at the mercy of the guides. Sometimes her lodging was an outhouse with the animals. Sometimes her escorts stole from her. One of her most heartrending experiences was when a particularly unpleasant guide insisted that she leave behind Petrus' diary and Bible. He said both were too dangerous to carry. She was forced to do as he said.

Strangely — or, perhaps, typically — this terrible journey didn't cause Susie to grow to dislike either the Tibetans or the Chinese. She knew that a woman travelling alone was defying all conventions, and that she couldn't really expect preferential treatment. Besides, many of her travelling companions were extremely kind to her, and so were some of the Chinese officials who sped her on her way. She met as much gallantry as cruelty. Nevertheless, it was with great relief that she reached China and eventually rode into the town of Ta-chien-lu (now K'ang-ting) where she knew there was a branch of the China Inland Mission. The night she entered the city, it was rocked by earthquake tremors — almost as if she were to be made to suffer every horror possible. But soon she was being welcomed into the mission house, being offered tea (in a *cup!*) and cookies, and a bath, and some fresh clothing — and such warming and kindly concern. At last she was truly among friends.

The first person who spoke to her at the mission, the first white man who had spoken to her since she last saw Petrus, was a missionary called Mr Moyes, and it is heartening to hear that, some years later, Susie became Mrs Moyes. She must have come to know Mr

Moyes well before she left China, for she spent six months at Ta-chien-lu, trying to discover what exactly had happened to Petrus and trying to track down his murderers. They were never caught, but they were discovered. They were discovered by Ishinima, the Kumbum lama who had taught the Rijnharts Tibetan. He was so upset when he heard the tragic story of the journey towards Lhasa that he set out alone to see if he could find any trace of Petrus.

So Susie returned to Canada to regain her health, to give lectures about Tibet, to write a book of her experiences and to drum up enthusiasm to send more missionaries to this hostile land. And before long, she herself was back in Tibet. Maybe it was the scene of her great tragedy, but it was a country she had grown to love.

Although Susie returned to Tibet for a few years, it was still known as Unoccupied Territory when she died in 1908.[8] But this is hardly surprising. Susie and Petrus had not been part of a great organization of missionaries: they had been trying to go it alone. They therefore had very little chance of establishing permanent and well-staffed hospitals and schools. They didn't have the facilities. Their achievement — and it was a most remarkable one — was that they did conduct a mission in Tibet, that they were able to preach the gospel in one of the greatest strongholds of Buddhism, that they made many friends, healed a great many people, and spread the gospel far into the interior. They left behind no monuments or institutions, but spiritually they achieved a great deal. They even half-converted a living Buddha.

However, their achievements do look rather pale when compared with the progress that was being made in neighbouring China. Around the turn of the century, hundreds of Canadians were working in China (as well, of course, as other nationalities) and many of them were medical missionaries. One organization alone — the Canadian Methodists' West China Mission — had recruited nearly a dozen of our women doctors by 1920 and had opened eleven hospitals, including a much-needed women's hospital, had established more than a hundred schools, numerous Bible training schools and a theological college, and had even started a Faculty of Medicine at the West China Union University (which was also missionary-sponsored).[9]

This was the pattern of missionary work throughout China — not only to convert and heal, but to train. Chinese women as well as men were trained to be teachers, nurses, *and* doctors, and in 1902 a medical assistant called Ah Mae Wong was sent all the way to Canada to study at the Ontario Medical College for Women. She graduated in 1906 and returned home to become one of the leading women physicians in Shanghai.[10]

All this makes heartening reading, but it was set against a background of terror and destruction. And the destruction wasn't wanton: it was the direct result of missionary behaviour. Susie Rijnhart had written: 'The work of Christian missions is hindered by antagonizing the non-Christian peoples through dogmatic assertion of doctrines and the failure of the Christian missionary to recognize and rejoice in the great underlying truths of all religions.'[11]

This was all too true. However liberal-minded our missionary doctors might be (and a good many of them were), they found that the non-Christian peoples had already been antagonized. Too many of the earlier missionaries had not been prepared to rejoice in underlying truths. Too many had rejoiced by burning idols, by ostentatiously eating meat in communities where vegetarianism was an article of faith, or by preaching against the theatre — regardless of the fact that wandering troupes of players were as much a part of daily life in China as television sets are in Canada today. In addition, few of the early Victorian missionaries seem to have felt much affection for the Chinese. They loved mankind, as they were bidden to do, but it was a curiously abstract form of love which didn't prevent them from despising the individuals they had been sent to convert.

Most of our medical missionaries arrived just in time for the backlash from this intolerant and unimaginative proseletyzing. China had had enough. Its hatred of foreigners — of all foreigners — had become obsessive, for while the missionaries had so singlemindedly been trying to Conquer China for Christ, their compatriots had been trying to conquer China for commerce, encroaching farther and farther into the heart of the Empire. Our eager young graduates from Toronto and Kingston could hardly have chosen a worse time to begin their life's work. First of all they were swept up in the anti-foreign riots of 1895; then there was the Boxer Rising of 1900, and then the revolution in 1911.

All were accompanied by violence and by the massacre of foreigners. During the Boxer Rising alone, 135 missionaries were slaught-

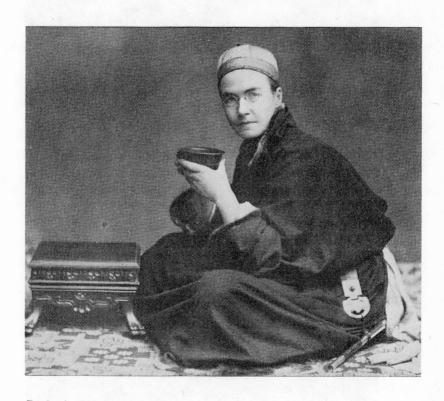

Dr Susie Rijnhart in Tibet

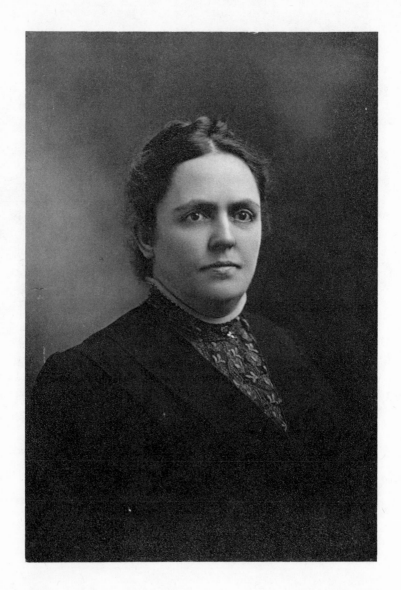

Dr Pearl Chute

ered[12] together with their children and converts, hacked down in their homes or herded into buildings which were set on fire. In Shansi Province, near Peking, forty-five men, women and children were rounded up and systematically beheaded, the children being killed while they were still holding their mothers' hands. Throughout the Empire, missionaries were attacked and mission property was destroyed. They were ordered to the coast and out of the country by their consuls, but it wasn't at all easy to get to the coast and they were liable to be killed, or at least attacked, on the journey.

In spite of the long journey to the coast, those farthest inland were sometimes the safest. Dr Alfretta Gifford Kilborn, a member of the West China Mission, survived as much because of the remoteness of the mission as because of the popularity of her medical work. The West China Mission was in Szechwan Province, far from the centre of the troubles, and although the Imperial decree to kill all foreigners arrived three weeks before the missionaries left, none of them were harmed; and when they returned the following year, they found that their property had been carefully guarded in their absence. But they were exceptionally lucky. In Honan Province, nearer Peking, Dr Jean Isabel Dow[13] (a young woman from Fergus, Ontario) literally had to flee for her life, in spite of her excellent medical work. But she, too, survived to make a come-back. Adversity brightened the missionary flame, rather than damping it.

Women doctors who were called to India were at least spared this type of adversity for Queen Victoria was Empress of India and the subcontinent was firmly under European domination. The Indians were in no position to rise up and slaughter the invaders. Conquering for Christ was therefore a far less hazardous business. Nevertheless, death was as near to the Indian missionaries as it was to those who went to China — death from cholera, typhoid, plague and dysentery. Some never returned to their homeland; many were broken in health when they did return. But some of them lived on to give a full life of service.

As in China, medicine was used as a vehicle through which to spread word of the Great Physician, but although it was only a means to an end, its value would be hard to overestimate. In a country where women were carefully guarded against the prying eyes of men, hospitals staffed by women doctors provided the women of India with the chance of receiving medical attention for the first time. In a country regulated by a rigid caste system, the advent of missionary hospitals provided the outcastes with a similar opportunity. Virtually no medical work had been done among these two large sections of the community before the missionaries moved in. And that was not all. As in China, the missionaries trained as well as healed. Many of the women doctors practising in India today were educated at missionary medical colleges — and these colleges are still in existence. So are hundreds, possibly thousands of hospitals which were started back in the last century by zealous young doctors who had been called to serve the Lord in this land of disease.

At Akidu, on the east coast of Central India, there is today a busy hospital with more than a hundred beds, an operating theatre, one Canadian nurse, a great many Indian nurses, and four Indian doctors — three of whom are women. This is the Star of Hope Hospital and it owes its existence to a group of Canadian Baptists. It owes its origins to a young woman from the Niagara Peninsula: Dr Pearl Smith Chute.[14]

Pearl Chute was an 1895 Trinity graduate (via Toronto's Woman's Medical College) and she was typical of the missionaries who went to India. But in one respect she was not at all typical: she had been an intern at St Michael's in Toronto. This was most unusual. Canadian hospitals didn't take women interns. There was no accommodation for them, and anyway women doctors were still such a suspect breed that most hospitals didn't want to take them in. Although the Woman's Medical College could offer its students clinical instruction at three hospitals — Toronto General, St Michael's and the Hospital for Sick Children — that was all it could offer in the way of hospital training, and most women doctors had to be content with that; unless they chose to intern in the United States. But apparently the nursing Sisters at St Michael's felt sorry for Pearl Smith and they used their influence to get her taken in.

So the young Baptist trained with the Catholics before setting off to heal the Hindus and Moslems. Very nonconformist. So was the fact that Pearl was travelling towards most of her family, rather than away from them. Her mother had died long ago and her father was busy farming at St Catharines, but a good part of the family was either in India already or on its way there. Pearl's elder sister, a nurse, travelled with her as chaperone, and both her brother and fiancé had already been working in Central India for a couple of years. Pearl's brother, Dr Everett Smith, had inaugurated medical work in the mission, and Pearl's fiancé, the Reverend Jesse Chute, had intended to be a medical missionary too, but he decided there was no need once he became engaged to Pearl. His district of Akidu wouldn't need two doctors.

Pearl was therefore the only doctor in Akidu and, at first, she was also the only woman doctor in the entire mission. But she didn't intend to start her medical work immediately. First she would learn the language, she said, and only then, when she could really be useful, would she let it be known that she was a physician. A sensible plan, but an unsuccessful one. On the first night in her new home — about the second night of her honeymoon — she and Jesse heard unexpected noises on their verandah: a woman in labour. Without pausing to learn a single word of Telegu, young 'Mrs Dr Chute' tore open her packing cases of surgical equipment and performed the delivery. Her practice had begun.

Apart from occasional home leave, she was to carry on her work at Akidu for nearly forty years. They were happy, busy, constructive years, and very much in the pattern of women doctors who worked in India. There were few traumatic setbacks here. The story of medical missions in India is one of sure and steady progress — the gradual development of a whole network of hospitals from practically nothing.

In 1896, when Pearl Chute began her medical work, there was no hospital in the district of Akidu. Her 'office' was her own verandah. The Chutes lived in a spacious, ex-army bungalow which was surrounded on all sides by a wide, shady verandah, so the office-and-dispensary was at least comparatively large. But it wasn't convenient for in-patients: even if Pearl had been sent to work among the sick, she didn't necessarily want them camping on her own verandah. But this situation didn't continue for long. The Baptists in Canada raised two hundred and thirty-five dollars, and this was more than enough to get Jesse Chute active. Like so many missionaries, he was an energetic builder: he built schools and churches throughout the district of Akidu, and he even built the chairs and blackboards. With more than two hundred dollars to spend on materials, it was no problem for him to build his wife a hospital.

Akidu's Star of Hope Hospital was opened in 1898 — a small

building among the palm trees. But it was a solid building of white-washed brick, with a strong red-tiled roof which could withstand even the heaviest rains. It had three rooms: a men's ward at one end, a women's ward at the other, and an office-dispensary-operating room decorously separating the two. The wards were always crowded: when a patient was hospitalized, the whole family moved in too, camping round the bed and doing the cooking outside the window. And the dispensary was as crowded as the wards. Pearl Chute was greatly admired, largely because of her medical work, but also because she was plump and had gold in her teeth; two sure signs of beauty. The villagers couldn't keep away.

In spite of her renowned beauty and her invaluable medical work, Dr Chute was not popular among the large population of Moslems at Akidu, or among the high-caste Hindus. Not at first. This was because most of her patients — like most of her husband's converts — tended to be outcastes, the untouchables, the very lowest order. The missionaries were accused of upsetting the balance of society, of raising the masses above their station, giving them unmerited comforts and attentions — and teaching them to read and write of all things!

The high caste might disapprove of the missionaries, but they couldn't do much to stop them and, bit by bit, they came round. They wouldn't attend the hospital — that would be too much to ask — but they would call for Dr Chute's services when they were really ill. Obligingly she went and treated them in their own homes, for she recognized the caste system as an institution, even if she wasn't in sympathy with it. Her tact was appreciated and, naturally, her practice grew . . . and grew.

One of the reasons for the increasing success of Dr Chute's medical work was that it wasn't an isolated affair like that of the Rijnharts. If she couldn't perform an operation herself, she could hand the case over to her brother to deal with on one of his regular visits to Akidu. If she diagnosed leprosy, she could send the patient up the coast to the mission's leper colony at Ramachandrapuram. There were sister hospitals not too far off and there was contact with sister as well as brother doctors — not only in the Baptist territory but in all the neighbouring provinces. And not far south, at Vellore, great things were taking place. The famous American missionary, Dr Ida Scudder, had started a hospital for women there, which soon developed into a medical school for female Indian Christians. Vellore was supported by a great many missions and by many different nations, and Dr Chute served on its board for some years.

The Chutes sent the most promising girls to Vellore to study and graduate in medicine, and by the time Pearl retired in 1930 many of the hospitals had at least one Indian woman on the staff. And of course there were Canadians too. Dr Chute had been the first woman doctor in the Baptist mission,[15] but she had soon been joined by others. In 1900, Dr Gertrude Hulet, a Trinity graduate, had joined the mission and had begun practising to the south of Akidu. In 1906, she had been joined by Dr Jessie Allyn (also from Trinity). In 1920, the Manitoba graduate, Bessie Findlay, had arrived. There were quite a number of women doctors working along the strip of coast that was Canadian Baptist territory.[16] But there was at least one whose work was soon over — Marjorie Cameron.

A cheerful and dedicated woman, Dr Cameron had joined the mission in 1915 and had taken over the management of the mission's Women's Hospital at Pithapuram. But she didn't hold the position for long. She was called to the Lord after only six years of service. Her death was alarmingly casual: she was taking a walk, and she just lay down and died.

Death in that steamy part of India could be as unexpected as it was sudden and yet Marjorie Cameron's death seems to have taken her colleagues by surprise. She didn't ail. She just went and died. However, the real surprise is not that Dr Cameron died but that so many of the others survived. Few of them escaped serious illness. Pearl Chute almost certainly had cholera — the symptoms were right — but she managed to struggle through. It was almost impossible to avoid infection, however careful you were. The Chutes took every possible precaution, eating only cooked food, drinking boiled water or 'hand milk' (the cow would be brought to the bungalow and milked while they watched, so that no canal water could be added to the pail), and yet cholera struck nonetheless. There was too much disease around and too little public health. A continual source of infection were the canals and stagnant, village ponds, which were used for everything from buffalo-washing to teeth-cleaning. Dr Chute did her best to encourage the villagers to dig wells — Jesse had dug her a well — but well water wasn't at all popular: it had no taste.

In spite of her bout of cholera, in spite of her exposure to a horrifying selection of skin complaints, to leprosy and almost every known tropical disease, Dr Chute managed to survive her years in India. She survived to give birth to five children, to see most of them grow up and follow her into medical or missionary work. She survived to see her small hospital replaced by a solid stone building and to see it staffed almost entirely by Indians. She survived to see the full fruit of her labours, and to be rewarded for them.

She had never been rewarded financially: she had not received any salary. Single women were paid by the mission, but wives of missionaries were expected to give their services free. Even though Pearl Chute charged her patients a small fee, these contributions went to the hospital, not to herself. In any case, the donations weren't very large. Dr Chute charged what a patient could afford — a handful of rice if he was poor, a handful of rupees if he was rich — just so that a value would be put on her work. In Akidu, something for nothing meant that the something was worth nothing.

Dr Chute therefore had very little material reward for her long life of service, but she had other more enduring rewards: affection and gratitude from the people of Akidu. And she received formal honours too. Before she died, she was awarded the Kaisar-i-Hind medal, a peculiarly Indian award which was bestowed only on people who had given outstanding service to the subcontinent. It is significant that at least half our women doctors who worked in India were honoured with the Kaisar-i-Hind.

While so many women doctors gave outstanding service to India, others served with a very different race of Indians — the native people of Canada. For instance, when Dr Chute was working in far-flung Akidu, a young woman called Elizabeth Scott Matheson was starting her medical work in the far-flung northwest of Canada. And she was doing so in the same manner as Pearl Chute: as missionary wife, rather than as doctor in her own right.

Elizabeth Scott Matheson was very much in the tradition of Canadian women doctors. Like Charlotte Ross, she braved driving snow and blistering sun in order to make her 'house calls'. Like Charlotte Ross, her medical education was a long-drawn-out process, interrupted and handicapped by the birth of children. Like Emily

Stowe, she had difficulty getting licensed. Like Emily Stowe, she practised for several years without a licence. Like Pearl Chute, she practised unpaid, in the role of missionary wife. Like Pearl Chute, she brought medical attention, for the first time, to the female Indians. And like many who both preceded and followed her, she lived to a great age and continued to work until she was well into her seventies.

Dr Elizabeth Scott Matheson was certainly true to type and yet she was uniquely herself. No other woman doctor brought up a family of between nine and a hundred children — depending on how you chose to count them. No other woman looked after such an outsized family while running a practice which covered a radius of more than a hundred miles. And no other woman found herself in the incongruous position of being appointed government doctor and health inspector when she was still being refused a licence by the College of Physicians and Surgeons. (In 1901 the government recognized her as the district's doctor, even though the College of Physicians and Surgeons refused to recognize her as any type of doctor). Was her position legal or illegal? In the northwest, along the North Saskatchewan river, nobody minded what it was. Deeds were more important than regulations, and it was by her deeds that Dr Matheson was recognized.

MISSIONARIES WHO SERVED IN CHINA

MARY ALFRETTA GIFFORD KILBORN (Trinity, 1891)

Retta Gifford (Mrs Kilborn) was the first medical woman to serve with the West China Mission — the Canadian Methodist mission that was established in the Province of Szechwan. She was the second wife of the mission's leader, Dr Omar Kilborn. His first wife had died of cholera only two months after arriving in Szechwan, but Retta Kilborn was more fortunate and she worked for many years at Chengtu, in Szechwan, opening and running the hospital for women and children there, serving on the staff of the West China Union University, and conducting a number of campaigns: she campaigned among the Chinese against the practice of foot-binding, and she campaigned (successfully) among her fellow missionaries to get women admitted as medical students at the West China Union University. More than once, she and her husband were forced to flee the mission because of anti-foreign riots, but in spite of danger and disease, she survived to give a full life of service. She retired to Canada in 1933 and died in Toronto, aged 78, in 1942.

JANET McCLURE KILBORN (Toronto, 1920)

Janet McClure married Retta Kilborn's eldest son. She was the daughter of one of the pioneers of the Canadian Presbyterian Mission in Honan, North China, and had been brought up in China. She served in Szechwan in the hospitals and in the university. She died in 1945.

JEAN DOW (Toronto, 1895)

Dr Dow was sent to Honan in North China in 1895, to succeed Dr Lucinda Graham who had recently died of cholera. For twenty years she was the only woman physician in the Canadian Presbyterian mission in Honan, but in 1918 she was joined by Dr Isabel McTavish, a Manitoba graduate. Both women were given medals by the Chinese for their work during the terrible famine of 1920-21. Dr Dow was well known in China for her work as a surgeon, but her greatest contribution was that she was among the first to isolate the organism which caused the very prevalent disease of Kola Azar. She died in Peking in 1927, at the age of 57.

JENNIE HILL MITCHELL (Trinity, 1895)

Jennie Hill (Mrs Mitchell) served in the Province of Honan with the American Presbyterian Church. She worked in China for more than 40 years.

MAUDE KILLAM NEAVE (New York, 1895)
Maude Killam (Mrs Neave) was a Maritimer who married a missionary and
served at Chengtu. She died there, of pneumonia, in 1920.

MABEL CASSIDY MORTIMER (Trinity, 1902) and MARTHA PHILP
BRADSHAW (Dalhousie, 1902)
Mabel Cassidy (Mrs Mortimer) and Martha Philp (Mrs Bradshaw) also
worked at Chengtu for the West China Mission.

JESSIE McBEAN (Toronto, 1905)
Dr McBean did most of her work in South China in hospitals at Macao,
Kongmoon and Canton.

MISSIONARIES IN MANY PLACES

KATE MacKAY MACKENZIE (Dalhousie, 1895)

Kate MacKay did her missionary work in Honolulu. She married
J.R. Mackenzie when she was home on leave and settled with him at
Edmonton, and then at Port Coquitlam, B.C. where she carried on a general
practice.

MARY IRWIN RUTNAM (Trinity, 1896)

Mary Irwin (Mrs Rutnam) went straight to Ceylon after her graduation, and
spent the rest of her life there. She worked as a doctor in Colombo, became
its first woman municipal councillor, and was very active in founding women's
institutes. She was decorated with the Ramón Magsaysay award for her
public service.

MARGARET STIRLING WALLACE (Trinity, 1898)

Dr Wallace was a medical missionary in both China and India. Driven from
her mission at Honan during the Boxer Rising, she worked for a short time
at a British Naval hospital — as a nurse, since the navy couldn't employ a
woman as a doctor. Later, she was transferred to India, where she was appointed
Vice-Principal at the Ludhiana Christian Medical College for Women.

ANNA HENRY (Trinity, 1898)

After serving in China and Japan for 30 years, mostly at Chengtu in West
China, Dr Henry went to Vancouver where she did missionary work among
the Chinese and Japanese in the city.

FLORENCE MURRAY (Dalhousie, 1919)

Dr Murray was a missionary in Manchuria and then in Korea from 1921 to
1969. She set up and ran hospitals, acted as surgeon, as public health officer,
taught in the medical school, trained nurses and interns, and also worked
among the lepers. A prolific writer, with a deep affection for Korea,
Dr Murray has written many articles about her medical work and about her
experiences during the Second World War.
An earlier Maritimer also worked as a missionary in Korea. This was
Dr KATE MacMILLAN of Jacquet River, N.B., a U.S. graduate, who started
her work in Korea in a two-room mud house. She died of typhus which she
contracted while caring for Korean schoolgirls during an epidemic of the
disease.

SIX MISSIONARIES TO INDIA

MARGARET O'HARA (Queen's, 1891)

Margaret O'Hara had four great loves: the Presbyterian Church, Queen's University, the British Empire, and India. She served all of these with faithful devotion during the 35 years she worked as a medical missionary at Dhar, near Indore. Apparently the training school, which she started for Indians at her hospital there, was based on the traditions of Queen's University. Queen's honoured her with an LL D for her long and valuable service in India, and she was also awarded the Kaisar-i-Hind medal. Besides being doctor, teacher, missionary, and one of Queen's most distinguished graduates, Dr O'Hara was also an author, writing a great many articles as well as the popular book *Leaves of the Lotus*. She died in Canada in 1940 at the age of 85.

LOUISA HELENA HART (New York, 1894)

Dr Hart was born in Shelburne, N.S. In 1944 she was awarded an honorary LL D by Mount Allison University. She spent much of her time in India working at the women's medical college at Vellore. She was decorated with the Kaisar-i-Hind medal and bar.

JESSIE ALLYN (Trinity, 1904)

Dr Allyn worked for many years with the Canadian Baptist Mission in Central India. She was responsible for starting the Women's Hospital at Pithapuram and she, too, was decorated with the Kaisar-i-Hind medal. On her retirement, she was appointed Secretary to the Christian Medical Association of India, Burma and Ceylon.

MARGARET PATTERSON (North-Western, 1899)

Another Kaisar-i-Hind medalist was Ontario-born Dr Patterson, who was decorated for her courageous work in Allahabad during a terrible epidemic of the bubonic plague. After her return to Canada, Dr Patterson was appointed as a magistrate — one of the first women ever to hold such a position. She died in 1963, aged 88.

ISABELLA THOMSON DAVIDSON (Trinity, 1902)

Isabella Thomson (Mrs Davidson) spent nearly 40 years as a missionary in Central India, doing much of her work with orphan children. She retired to Scarborough, her family town (Dr Davidson's great-grandparents had been its first settlers).

MILDRED JEAN HOYLES HASLAM (Toronto, 1903)
Jean Hoyles (Mrs Haslam) was appointed as a missionary for the Anglican Church of Canada. She worked at Kangra, in the very north of India, where she established the Maple Leaf Hospital for women and children.

7

Women and children first

ALTHOUGH Elizabeth Scott Matheson worked much of her life in the secondary role of missionary wife, she was a missionary before her husband ever was.[1] When she first met John Matheson, he was a rip-roaring trapper cum trader, cum guide, cum adventurer, cum just about everything in the West, a boisterous and high-spirited man who enjoyed drinking and card-playing and who seems to have been something of an embarrassment to his relatives. John's brother was the Reverend Edward Matheson and his cousin was the Reverend Samuel Matheson, who later became Archbishop of Rupert's Land and Primate of All Canada. John was not the family black sheep — he was far too likeable — but he was hardly a suitable husband for young Elizabeth Scott, and he courted her for six years before she agreed to marry him.

Elizabeth was teaching in Manitoba when she first came to know John Matheson. She had been born near Campbellford, Upper Canada, in 1866, but her family had moved west and it was in Winnipeg that she attended high school and trained to be a teacher. She was a sprightly young woman, but serious and with a true sense of vocation, and when she left Manitoba in 1887, it was to take on volunteer work in a home for orphans. This was followed by one year at the Women's Medical College in Kingston and then by a seven year contract with a Presbyterian mission in India. There seemed little likelihood that she would ever see Matheson again, but fortunately for him — and also for Saskatchewan — Elizabeth caught malaria in India and she was sent home, ill but alive, to Canada.

In the meantime, John Matheson had had a change of heart. Having spread his activities to include railway construction, prospecting and mining, he was well on his way to becoming a building contractor when he attended a revivalist meeting — and discovered his true vocation. It seems to have been one of those sudden conversions. There was no doubt in his mind: he knew that he had been called to serve the Lord.

Surprisingly, John's clerical relatives were not too pleased when they heard this news. They were uncertain of John's sincerity. He had tried his hand at so many different professions . . . surely this was just another of his wild schemes. Certainly it did seem out of character, but John gradually managed to convince his relatives that this was no passing whim, so they agreed to help him and in 1892 they got him appointed as missionary to an Indian reserve at Onion Lake, on the understanding that he would study for the priesthood and serve as an Anglican clergyman.

It was not exactly a plum job. Onion Lake, up near Fort Pitt on the northern arm of the Saskatchewan River, was barely on the map in 1892. Only twenty-five years had passed since the Hudson's Bay Company had sold the vast area of Rupert's Land to the Federal Government, and although this area was now known as Canada's North-West Territories and was open to settlement, very few homesteaders had crept far northwards yet. In fact one could say that most of the North-West Territories (the whole of the Canadian north and west apart from Manitoba and British Columbia) were nothing much except territory. Only in the south had there been any very populous settlement: a rapid growth along the line of the railway. And although there were a few quite large communities to the north of the main east-west line, Onion Lake was certainly not one of them. There was almost nothing at Onion Lake: one Hudson's Bay Company post, a small detachment of the North-West Mounted Police, a Roman Catholic mission, a Protestant mission and the odd trader and trapper. That was about the sum total of the white presence.

Both the Catholic and Protestant missions had been set up at Onion Lake shortly after the reserves had been established there in 1876, and the Catholic mission had been doing quite well because of all the Métis settlements clustered around the reserves.

But the Anglicans had made little progress. There was only one Indian family that was nominally Anglican; the mission school was a small and deserted log cabin, the mission church was a small and deserted lop-sided building that looked as if it was about to fall over, and the mission 'residence' was little more than a four-roomed hut. It was enough to deter the most zealous, especially as the salary that accompanied this unenviable appointment was only three hundred dollars a year. But John Matheson was not at all dismayed. He approached his new appointment with the zest of an overseas missionary entering an Unoccupied Field. 'I earned a good living serving the devil,' he announced firmly. 'I can earn a better one serving the Lord.'

It wasn't long before he was doing so.

When John set off for Onion Lake in 1892, he was accompanied by his bride — Elizabeth had at last agreed to marry him. Even if John had not been deeply in love with Elizabeth, he could hardly have chosen a more suitable partner. Elizabeth was not a doctor at this time — she had only done one year of medicine — but at least she had some medical knowledge, and she was also a fully qualified teacher, which was considered more to the point. For this was to be a teaching mission. The Métis and Treaty Indians of the area were to be Christianized through education rather than through medicine. John had been a teacher as a young man, so he too had teaching experience, but more important, he had long experience of relying on his own resources in the northwest. He could speak French, he was fluent in Cree, and he already had a great many Indian friends. He was also a very practised trader.

This was to serve him well, for three hundred dollars a year was not enough for the type of mission he wanted to establish. Before long he took up trading again — as a sideline to his pastoral work — taking seneca root and furs to Edmonton each spring and returning with enough supplies to see the mission through another year. In addition, he started a cattle ranch, a farm and gardens, and he built stables and storehouses. In fact, he ran the mission as a form of self-supporting business. And he built. How he built!

His first building project was to prop up the church, but soon he was adding rooms to his house, then more rooms, another wing, and even a three-storey schoolhouse. Part of the reason for all this building activity was the Mathesons' growing family. Elizabeth had become pregnant very soon after her marriage, but she was only to give birth to nine of her children. The rest, the other eighty or so, were gathered in, taken in almost casually. The couple had already added about twelve Indian children to their family by the end of their first winter.

It was the Mathesons' school which caused them to acquire such a large family. The first classes had been very poorly attended — there would be just a handful of children, sometimes none, for the Indian people didn't feel that it was particularly important that their children should go to school every day. So the Mathesons began to board the pupils in their own home, building on rooms as they were required. Children who had no parents were adopted, and others were simply fostered for ten years or so, but all were considered part of the family and most of them were fed, clothed and housed at the Mathesons' expense.

The Mathesons could get a small government grant for each Treaty Indian who was taken in, but most of the children were Métis from outside the reserve and they weren't provided with a grant. Nor, of course, were white children, though the parents of white children could sometimes contribute to their support. The white children grew in numbers as the years passed because this was the only real school in the area, so families living as much as seventy miles away would send their children to Onion Lake. The Matheson family was therefore an inter-racial group, although the Métis predominated. It was also inter-denominational. John was an Anglican clergyman, Elizabeth was Presbyterian — and some of their children were Roman Catholics. Nobody was refused admission to this large and happy family.

It was the size of her family which induced Elizabeth to return to medical school — or, rather, which induced John to send her back to school: she wasn't very keen to go. Elizabeth was enjoying her work at Onion Lake and she didn't want to be separated for three years or so either from her children or from her magnificent husband. Besides, she had already conceived her third child — although John didn't know this at the time. Typically, Elizabeth didn't tell him. John had already raised the money for her fees and had secured a teacher for the school. And there was no doubt that the mission did need a doctor: there was no physician nearer than Battleford, a hundred miles away. So Elizabeth set off for Winnipeg to enrol as a second year student at the Manitoba Medical College.

The Manitoba Medical College had been established in 1883, and it had never officially *not* accepted women. Already it had graduated its first woman doctor. This was Harriet Foxton Clarke who had done her first two years at the Toronto Woman's Medical College and her final years at Manitoba.[2] The precedent was therefore established both in accepting a woman student and in recognizing the exams she had taken at a women's college. So although it was seven years since Elizabeth had sat first year medicine at Kingston, her work there was recognized without opposition — and so was her presence in a 'mixed' class at Manitoba Medical College. No male onslaught awaited her, no scribbles on the wall or sniggers in the classroom. In fact, when Elizabeth decided to withdraw from the course, because of her pregnancy, the acting dean was extremely upset. Why was she leaving? Had any of the students been unpleasant to her?

Elizabeth laughed.

'But, Dr Jones, I thought you would know why I'm withdrawing,' she said. 'After all, your field is obstetrics.'

Dr Jones seems to have taken this revelation in his stride, and instead of railing against the impossibility of trying to educate women, he insisted on delivering Elizabeth's baby himself.

In spite of Dr Jones' support, Elizabeth's final student years were not taken in Manitoba — she was to attend *three* different colleges before she graduated. This was because a friend of John Matheson's offered to pay her fare to Toronto: it would be much more pleasant for her to study with other women, he said. So off went Elizabeth to the Ontario Medical College for Women, but not in the best of health. She had developed mastitis after the birth of her child and she was so obviously unwell when she arrived in Toronto that a message was sent to John asking him to use his influence to get her to return home. The answer John sent back was very typical, and it pleased nobody except Elizabeth: 'No man, having put his hand to the plough, and looking back, is fit for the Kingdom of God.'

Encouraged by her husband, Elizabeth kept her hand firmly on the plough, sat her second and third year exams in one year, and graduated MD CM from Trinity in 1898. It had taken her eleven years to graduate, but, like Emily Stowe, this wasn't the end of her struggles: it was only the beginning.

Elizabeth's Trinity degree qualified her for registration in Ontario, but it didn't qualify her in the North-West Territories. An earlier Trinity graduate, Etta Denovan, had only been registered in the North-West Territories after she had sat a local exam.[3] This was normal policy — similar to the regulations in the east — and it had not been difficult for Dr Denovan to comply: she was living in Calgary at the time and the North-West Territories registration examinations were generally held in Calgary. But Calgary was a long and expensive distance from Onion Lake, and in any case, Elizabeth didn't want to sit the exam. She was sure it was an oral, and she had heard of trick questions being asked. She had also heard (perhaps erroneously) that certain male graduates from Trinity had not been made to sit the oral. So she applied for registration without offering to take the exam. And, of course, she was refused.

This was of no great importance up at Onion Lake. Most of Elizabeth's patients were likely to be members of the mission — her own children — and they weren't going to quibble about her qualifications. More important to Elizabeth, and more of a drawback to her work, was that nobody at Onion Lake really recognized her as a doctor: in spite of her degree, she was still thought of as Mrs. Matheson, the missionary's wife. The few whites in the district continued to manage on their own, or — in severe emergencies — to travel all the way to Battleford to consult the doctor there. The Indians continued to consult their own medicine men. And the mission children remained remarkably healthy. After all that effort and all those years of study, Elizabeth found herself with nothing to do. There wasn't even much to do around the mission, for the staff had increased while she was away and everything was running smoothly. She even seemed to have lost her role as mother. Her own children had been separated from her for so long that they turned to others when they wanted affection or attention. It was not an auspicious beginning.

Elizabeth was not called out on her first real case until 1899, a year after she had graduated and very shortly after she had given birth to her fourth child. The Indian Agency cattle had been driven

into the bush country for the winter, seventy-five miles northwest
of Onion Lake and the son of the cattleman had broken his leg.
A telegram was sent to the mission asking the doctor to come immediately.

The reaction to the telegram was one of outrage. How could this
man expect Mr Matheson's wife to travel so far in such weather?
Although there was no snow yet, the frost was hard on the ground,
and it was monstrous to subject Mrs Matheson to such conditions.
Why, she was still nursing her baby! What could the man be
thinking of?

'He is thinking that I am the doctor,' said Elizabeth firmly.

'That's my Bess!' said John Matheson proudly. *He* hadn't been
outraged by the call for help, and immediately he set about planning the journey — she would need to keep the baby well wrapped
up, and she should have plenty of furs for herself, and who would
be best to send along as driver?

A short while later Dr Elizabeth Matheson set off courageously
on her first case — seventy-five miles in a heavy lumber wagon across
frozen ground, with a young man as driver and her own tiny baby
in a moss-bag in her arms. It took her two days to reach her patient,
and three days to return, with a harsh homeward journey through
a heavy snowstorm. But she arrived home triumphant. She had
done it! She had proved that she really was a doctor — proved it
to herself as well as to the people of Onion Lake.

From then on, she never looked back. John built her a three-
storey hospital, complete with operating room; the local whites
began to turn to her for treatment, and the Indian people began
to do so too. She was fully recognized as the Onion Lake doctor.
Within a few years she even received an official appointment: Onion
Lake was hit by a smallpox epidemic in 1901 — there were forty
cases in the school alone — and Elizabeth's work in coping with the
epidemic came to the attention of the Department of Indian Affairs.
As a result, she was appointed government doctor to the Indians,
with a salary of three hundred dollars a year — regardless of the
fact that she still had no licence to practise.

This was unimportant as far as Onion Lake was concerned. The
Mounties continued to help Elizabeth in whatever way they could
and to consult her professionally, and the few homesteaders who
were moving into the area consulted her too. After all, if you broke

your leg so far away from any settlement or city, you were only too glad to find someone who knew how to set it.

But the character of Onion Lake was changing, and it changed dramatically in 1903 when the Barr colony was established only thirty-five miles away at Lloydminster. Suddenly there were thousands of people in the neighbourhood. One of the Barr colonists was a physician,[4] and it wasn't long before others were also setting up a practice in Lloydminster. Elizabeth's irregular position was no longer tenable so once again she applied for a licence. But since she still refused to sit the exam, her registration was again refused. An additional problem was that Elizabeth didn't think she would pass the exam now, even if she agreed to take it. Although she had been practising busily as a doctor, her practice had been limited to the requirements of her patients, and she was out of touch with some of the subjects she would be examined on. So she decided to go back to medical school and take her final year again.

This time she got her degree from the University of Manitoba; it was the nearest medical school. And as there wasn't one in Calgary — or anywhere in the North-West Territories — surely the NWT Registrar would recognize its degree. Just to make sure, Elizabeth registered herself in Manitoba as soon as she had graduated there in 1904. But the Registrar remained firm. No exam, no licence.

By this time John Matheson had had enough. Angrily he wrote out a cheque for her registration fee. 'Send it off to them,' he said. Elizabeth did so, and to her great surprise, received her registration by return mail. Why? Why this sudden change of policy? The only explanation was John Matheson's name on the cheque, a name that had become famous throughout the North-West. Elizabeth was no longer just another of those difficult women. She was the wife of the famous missionary, John Matheson.

Elizabeth didn't mind being cast as missionary wife. She was no feminist and she didn't demand recognition for her own performance. She was extremely humble about her work, insisting that she was doing no more than any other pioneering woman. Yet her humility was blended with a firmness which at times amounted to obstinacy. After all, the long struggle for registration had been the result of her own intransigence — it wasn't entirely the fault of 'male man'. Maybe she was humble, but she wasn't meek. She was a

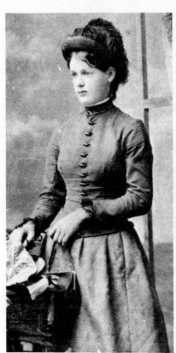
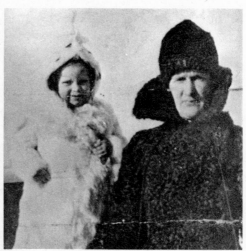
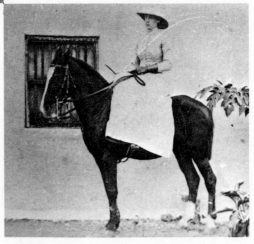

Dr Elizabeth Scott Matheson as a school teacher in Manitoba, 1883-87 (left); as a missionary in India, 1889-90 (below right) and with her daughter, Ruth, at Onion Lake, 1909 (above right)

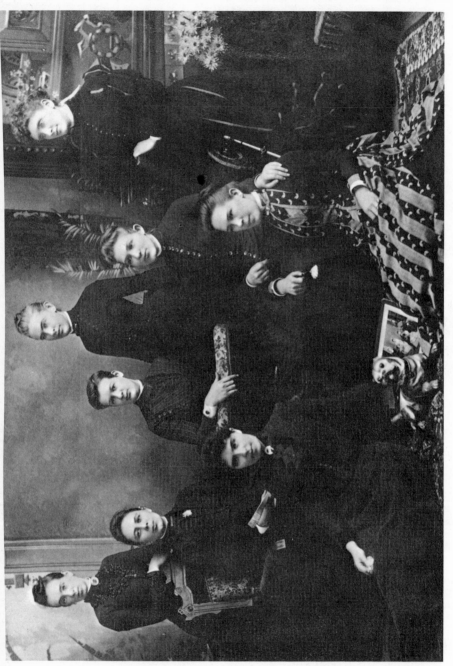

Class photo, Women's Medical College, Kingston, 1887-88
Standing (left to right): Janet Murray, Margaret O'Hara, Nellie Skimmen
Seated: Janet Weir, Elizabeth Scott (Matheson), Jean Sinclair

very warm person, but brisk, purposeful, pragmatic, humorous, admired as much as loved, and always respected.

She gained respect very early on, and not only for her medical work. From the beginning, she had been her husband's equal partner in the mission and when John Matheson became ill towards the end of his life, Elizabeth took over most of the administration of the school — as well as continuing her medical practice and as well as being mother to her many children. Where her children were concerned, she was always ready to defend, or even attack. On one occasion she rounded on a settler's wife who had wandered into the mission with her small child — a small child who had a most recognizable cough.

'That child has whooping-cough!' said Dr Matheson accusingly. 'Whooping-cough — and you've brought her here among all my children. You had no *right* to do such a thing!'

Alarmed at this sudden attack, the settler's wife mumbled an apology. . . . Very sorry . . . didn't know you had any children (surely all these missionaries were spinsters).

'I have one hundred children,' announced Dr Matheson — and marched off indignantly, her anger turning to laughter as she wondered how the poor woman was going to work that one out.

Certainly Dr Matheson thought of all the children as her own. They were brought up as one family in the Mathesons' house, which became a large boarding school. Elizabeth never had a home that was truly her own until she left Onion Lake after her husband had died.

That was the end of an era for her. John Matheson died in 1916, and although Elizabeth carried on the mission for another year, acting as school principal and as both parents as well as resident doctor, her work at Onion Lake was drawing to its close. In 1917 a new principal was appointed and the Church assumed full responsibility for the school. So the Matheson home was no longer needed, not officially at any rate.

Elizabeth was fifty years old at this time, still very vigorous, still the humble authoritarian, still strong in her sense of duty and not at all ready to retire. She could have chosen to work almost anywhere in Canada — she was qualified in most provinces — but she chose Winnipeg because she was offered a job there.

When Elizabeth took up her work in Winnipeg in 1918, the

Yeomans ladies had been gone some time, but there were two
women practising in the city: Dr Mary Crawford and Dr Edith
Ross, the granddaughter of Charlotte Ross. In addition there was
Dr Ellen Douglass, who had gone overseas for the war and had not
yet returned. Winnipeg really had three women doctors. Of these
three, Mary Crawford was the leader, the oldest, the most well-
known. For some years, she had been acting as medical inspector of
public schools and it was she who invited Elizabeth Matheson to
Winnipeg. Dr Crawford was the only doctor giving medical examinations to schoolchildren, and she could do with an assistant of
Elizabeth Matheson's calibre.

Dr Crawford was a stern, rather formal woman, with a presence
that didn't encourage intimacies, but apparently she was very gentle
with the children — a common bond with Dr Matheson. The two
women were to become close friends, although they were never on
Christian-name terms (somehow you couldn't call Dr Crawford
'Mary') and they worked harmoniously together for many years.
Elizabeth didn't retire from being school inspector until she was
seventy-five.

Of course, she was ideally suited to the work. Most of her practice had been among poor children — the Indian children of the
mission — and she was quick to recognize signs of malnutrition or
symptoms of the many 'children's diseases'. She could hardly have
found a more suitable position, or one that was more worthwhile.

The medical inspection of schoolchildren was a public health
measure, which had been started in Montreal in 1906,[5] and it was
immensely valuable. How valuable could be seen from the results,
for as many as half the school children examined were found to need
medical attention. With most of them, this was the first time they
had ever been seen by a doctor. Decaying teeth, enlarged tonsils,
weak eyesight as well as more serious complaints were corrected
through this survey, and the mentally retarded and slow learners
also received special attention and were often given separate
classes. The school inspectors acted as welfare officers as much as
physicians, following their patients from school to home, and finding out why some children didn't attend school. Often it was because they lacked clothing and were too proud to go to school in
rags, and in such cases clothes were provided for them.

A great many of our women doctors were appointed school inspectors, partly because this was considered suitable work for them, and partly because it was one of the few openings available. For women still had very little opportunity in medicine. If they didn't want to be missionaries or pioneers, they really had to settle for work with women or children. Most other branches of the profession were firmly closed against them.

In spite of this they were gaining ground and, for a few of them, appointments as school inspectors led to far more prestigious appointments. One woman medical inspector not only gained a position on the staff of the Toronto General Hospital, but was appointed head of child welfare for the Federal Government. This was Dr Helen MacMurchy, a University of Toronto graduate (MB 1900, MD 1901), an outstandingly brilliant woman and one of the giants of the profession.

From the very beginning, Dr MacMurchy's achievements were exceptional. At Toronto she won first class honours in medicine and surgery, she actually managed to intern at the Toronto General Hospital — said to be the first woman to do so — and then went on to take postgraduate work at the Johns Hopkins Hospital in Baltimore.[6] Then for seven years she was Ontario's provincial inspector of hospitals, prisons and charitable institutions, as well as being Secretary to the Canadian Medical Association's committee on the medical inspection of schools.

Very early in her life, Dr MacMurchy had become a well-known public figure, writing careful and detailed reports to the CMA *Journal,* delivering lectures, presenting medical papers, writing books on motherhood and on the care of infants — and also becoming the first editor of the *Canadian Nurse* journal.[7] When, in 1920, she was appointed to take charge of the Federal Government's Division of Child Welfare,[8] few people can have been very surprised. And yet it was most unusual for a woman to be given quite such a responsible government post. But then Dr MacMurchy was extremely unusual: before she died, she was named one of the ten leading women physicians in the entire western world.

Her most important contribution to medicine was in mother-and-child welfare, rather than simply child welfare, and this was her chief concern in her work with the government. At the beginning of this century, not only was the infant mortality rate desperately high, but the mothers were dying too — of puerperal sepsis. That was why Dr MacMurchy published books on motherhood and on the care of infants. That was why she lectured so widely. It was all part of her public health campaign to reduce the death rate and to allow the population of Canada to grow as it was felt it should grow. During her years with the Federal Government, Dr MacMurchy achieved a very marked decline in the death rate from puerperal sepsis. Many more mothers survived to give birth to further children — and their children survived too.

But while Dr MacMurchy's first concern was to ensure that the children who were born would survive to become adults, a related concern was naturally birth control. It was the health of the mother and the health of the family as a whole that mattered — too many children weren't always desirable — so while, on the one hand, Dr MacMurchy was writing special reports on Infant Mortality, on the other hand she was issuing booklets on Family Planning. It wasn't as contrary as it might seem. It was all part of the same program. So, too, was the care of the mentally retarded. This was another area of medicine which was gaining increasing attention and which was especially gaining the attention of women doctors.

Throughout the country, women were moving into the field of mental as well as physical health. In Winnipeg for instance, Dr Matheson's associate, Mary Crawford, was doing a great deal for the mentally retarded as part of her school inspection work, and far away in the east of Canada there was another woman doctor working in the same field. This was Dr Eliza Perley Brison,[9] a graduate from Dalhousie University. Dr Brison was herself handicapped, physically handicapped — she had had her hip joint removed when she was in her early twenties — and although this caused her to withdraw from medicine from time to time, it didn't prevent her from initiating a new and sympathetic approach to the care of the mentally retarded. Until she started her work in the Maritimes, very little had been done there for the mentally retarded. For the most part, they were regarded as lost causes or as semi-human, and the main purpose in putting them into institutions had been to protect society from them, rather than to help them in any way.

Dr Brison took a totally different approach. 'Better a disciplined moron than an undisciplined genius,' was her tenet. But the discipline had to be kindly. She left one girls' home in New Brunswick because a new director was appointed, who insisted on using force and putting the girls into strait jackets. This was contrary to all Dr Brison's beliefs. Kindness, gentleness and understanding were the tools of her trade, and very successful they were too. Under her gentle guidance, she succeeded in helping a great many patients to live comparatively purposeful and creative lives — and certainly much happier lives than they had lived before they came under her care.

At first, most of her patients were women and children, as they were bound to be, but at the age of fifty she was appointed psychiatrist for Nova Scotia's Department of Health and Welfare. This was in 1931, eleven years after Dr MacMurchy had received her appointment with the Federal Government, and at a time when women were beginning to be accepted in all branches of medicine.

However, there were still not many women psychiatrists. Dr Brison had studied psychiatry after leaving Dalhousie, taking a postgraduate course in the United States, and in fact many of her innovations were the result of treatment she had seen being given in the States. But as many others were the result of her own personality. She was a strange mixture, very quiet, very kind and yet extremely determined. If she hadn't been so determined, she would never have surmounted her own handicap. It was this quiet determination, a gentle and almost unnoticeable persistence which brought her so much success with her patients.

For instance, it was typical that, of all the staff at the Welfare Office, it was only Dr Brison who managed to calm an alarmingly disturbed patient who burst in one day. He was large and he was frightened and he was also frightening, and the staff could do nothing to calm him. But then Eliza Brison came out of her office, hobbling slowly towards the man on her crutches. She looked at him sympathetically and without any alarm. 'You're disturbed,' she said sadly. His anger and panic evaporated immediately. Yes, he was indeed disturbed — at least he had been until Dr Brison appeared. Quietly he followed the lady doctor into her office to tell her the story of what had upset him.[10]

Dr Brison continued to work with the mentally retarded until she was well into her seventies, by which time similar work was being done in most of the mental institutions throughout Canada. For the work of physicians across the country was becoming closely connected, an interrelated part of a single development. This was a historical process, a result of the welding together of Canada as a nation. No longer did one look west expecting to find rather rough and ready medical work. The pioneering age was passing. And no longer did one necessarily have to look to Ontario or Quebec for the latest and newest developments in medicine.

Naturally one used to look east, and especially to French Canada for that was where it had all begun. Our first hospital was the Hôtel Dieu in Quebec which was founded as early as 1639.[11] Our first medical college was also founded in French Canada. This was the Montreal Medical Institution, the forerunner of McGill's Faculty of Medicine, which was opened in 1823. Even after Confederation, the Province of Quebec continued to lead the way and it wasn't surprising that the medical inspection of schoolchildren should have been started in Montreal.

But while French Canada was the first in the field in so many areas of medicine, it wasn't at all forward in promoting the cause of women in medicine. Maybe Dr Charlotte Ross had managed to practice in Montreal in the late 1870's, but she hadn't swept in a whole tide of women doctors. Until 1900 there were hardly any women practising medicine in the Province of Quebec. This was because there were no facilities for them: very little was offered in the way of education and even less in the way of encouragement. The women of Quebec weren't either expected or required to take up medicine. If they decided to do so, they were on their own and they would have to look elsewhere for their education. They would have to look a long way off if they were French speaking.

WOMEN OF THE WEST

HARRIET FOXTON CLARKE (Manitoba, 1892)
The first woman graduate from the Manitoba Medical College, Harriet Foxton (Mrs Clarke) had been born at Brockville, Ontario, and had started her medical studies in Toronto before moving to Winnipeg. After her graduation, she married Dr Andrew Clarke of Detroit, and practised in the United States.

MARGARET MacMILLAN FORSTER (Trinity, 1895)
One of the earliest medical women in the West was Margaret MacMillan (Mrs Forster) who practised in Victoria between 1896 and 1900. In 1900 she moved to New Westminster and then, in 1902, settled in Alberta. Of her three children, the two girls both took up medicine, the elder (Dr Sylling) as a physician and the younger as a nurse.

ANNIE VERTH JONES (Trinity, 1896)
Annie Verth (Mrs Jones) practised medicine in Rossland and Nelson, B.C. However, after ten years, her health failed, and she retired to Ontario.

MARGARET DOUGLAS FRENCH (Durham, 1904)
Dr French was born in England and graduated from Durham University. In Canada, she worked first at Shellbrook, where she was a medical health officer for 12 years and then she moved to Saskatoon where she practised until her retirement. She died in 1951 at the age of 73.

MARGARET GARDNER HOGG (Glasgow, 1904)
Margaret Gardner (Mrs Hogg) practised in Vancouver for many years and, for a time, worked for the city schools. She died as a result of a motor accident in 1930.

146

WOMEN DOCTORS IN WINNIPEG

MARY CRAWFORD (Trinity, 1900)

Mary Crawford was the daughter of a Scottish sea captain and a Scottish schoolmistress, and she came to Ottawa as a child when her mother was appointed principal of Ottawa Ladies' College. Mary was encouraged to follow her mother's profession, and pressure was put on her to train as a kindergarten teacher, but she was more interested in music and medicine, neither of which were considered suitable professions. It was only after her mother's death that Mary Crawford was able to enter medical school.

She was to become an extremely successful doctor and in 1930-31 she was appointed President of the Federation of Medical Women of Canada. By this time Dr Crawford had gained wide recognition for her work as medical inspector of Winnipeg's public schools. Dr Crawford also developed a special interest in the mentally retarded, and she introduced mental testing into the schools and organized special classes for the mentally handicapped.

MARGARET ELLEN DOUGLASS (Trinity, 1905)

Ellen Douglass was born in New Brunswick and she took a course at the University of New Brunswick before going on to Toronto to study medicine. After postgraduate training in the United States and England, she practised for a while in Saint John, N.B. and then moved to Winnipeg in 1909. In 1914 she organized the Winnipeg Women's Volunteer Reserve and, later in the war, she took a draft of VAD's to England. She served in France with the RAMC, holding the rank of major and she was awarded the Allies Medal and the British War Medal for her service. In 1919 she returned to Winnipeg and continued to practise there until her retirement. She died in 1950.

EDITH ROSS (Manitoba, 1913)

Edith Ross, granddaughter of Charlotte Whitehead Ross, was the first woman to practise as an anaesthetist at the Winnipeg General Hospital. She won the Gold Medal when she graduated from Manitoba Medical College in 1913 and she gained a reputation as an anaesthetist at both the Winnipeg General and St Boniface Hospital — in spite of the brevity of her career. She died in 1932 after a long illness.

WELFARE AND PUBLIC HEALTH

GERALDINE OAKLEY (Toronto, 1912)

Geraldine Oakley did so much for the children of Calgary that a school was
named after her: the Dr Oakley Junior High School. She was born in
Stratford, Ontario, and her early medical work was done in the east. In 1915,
when the Women's College Hospital and Dispensary was opened in Toronto
as a 21-bed hospital, Dr Oakley was appointed its medical superintendent.
She moved to Calgary in 1918 in order to take up the position of medical
inspector of Calgary's public schools (a position which had previously been
held by Dr Rosamond Leacock). From then on, Dr Oakley dedicated her life
to the health of the children of Calgary, holding regular clinics in all the
public schools and also running a baby clinic at the City Hall. In 1935, when
school and city health services were combined, Dr Oakley was appointed
Calgary's Assistant Medical Health Officer. She died in 1948.

MARGARET McALPINE (Toronto, 1905)

Margaret McAlpine worked for Toronto's health department for 35 years.
Born in Mount Forest, she was brought up in Collingwood and was educated
there before going to the Ontario Medical College for Women in Toronto.
After her graduation, she interned at the Woman's Hospital in Philadelphia.

MABEL LOUISE HANNINGTON (Toronto and Trinity, 1900)

Dr Hannington was a native of Saint John, N.B. and, after serving as a
missionary in China, she returned to New Brunswick where, in 1919, she was
appointed medical inspector of schools. By 1920 she had about 8000 children
under her supervision. In 1933-34 Dr Hannington held the position of
President of the Federation of Medical Women of Canada.

ANNIE ROSS (Trinity, 1902)

For many years Dr Ross was a house mother to the students at the Ontario
Agricultural College in Guelph; she also lectured to women students at the
Macdonald Institute until her retirement in 1936. She was an honorary
member of the St John Ambulance. She died in Goderich in 1966, aged 94.

ELIZA PERLEY BRISON (Dalhousie, 1911)

After graduating from Dalhousie, Dr Brison spent a year at North Hampton
State Hospital as a resident in psychiatry, and after a period of ill health
when she cared for mentally retarded children in her home, she registered

as a student at the Walter E. Fernald State School for the Mentally Deficient.
On returning to Canada, she became Superintendent of the IODE Home for
Girls in Halifax until it was closed in 1925. In 1929 she became an anaesthetist
at Victoria General Hospital — the first female doctor to be appointed to the
staff — and in 1931 she joined the staff of Nova Scotia's Department of Public
Health, becoming psychiatrist for the province. After her retirement,
Dr Brison continued to work for the mentally retarded as a consulting
psychiatrist and, on a number of occasions, as superintendent of homes for
the retarded. Dr Brison was awarded the Coronation Medal of Queen
Elizabeth II.

ELIZABETH KILPATRICK (Dalhousie, 1915)
Born in Cape Breton, Dr Kilpatrick took postgraduate work in the United
States. She too became a psychiatrist, and she practised in the United States
until she returned to Halifax in 1959 and took a teaching position in
psychiatry at Dalhousie University. She died in 1969 at the age of 77.

EDITH HAMILTON GORDON (Toronto, 1915)
After graduation, Dr Gordon did a year at Philipsburg Hospital, Pennsylvania,
and was then appointed assistant medical adviser of women students at
Cornell University. In 1920 she graduated from the University of Pennsylvania
with the degree of DPH and was appointed medical adviser to women at the
University of Toronto.

8

Montreal and Maude Abbott

IN THE last century, in fact almost until the middle of this century, there was nowhere in Canada where a French-Canadian woman could study medicine in her own language. Consequently there are few French names among our pioneers. The earliest is Madame Bruère who went all the way to Paris to study, graduating in 1891, but Madame Bruère may only have been French Canadian by marriage. Her maiden name was Elizabeth Walker. However, she returned to Canada and set up a practice in Montreal and she was working there in the 1890's in an office that she shared with her husband and fellow-physician, Andrew Arthman Bruère.[1] Some years later Irma LeVasseur was to graduate in Minnesota and return to Quebec to practise. She was thoroughly Quebecoise, but she was still at school in the 1890's. Her career hadn't begun yet. Meanwhile all the other French-Canadian women who were interested in medicine seem to have had to settle for being either nurses or midwives.

At first the situation was no better among the English-speaking communities in Quebec — except that would-be women doctors only had to travel as far as Kingston in order to get a degree in medicine in their own language. Yet they still had to go outside the province. McGill should have led the way — it had been the first Canadian university to establish a medical faculty — but it held out against taking women as medical students until 1918, more than a quarter of a century after Queen's had first accepted women. Even then it might not have changed its policy if it hadn't been for Dr Maude Elizabeth Seymour Abbott.[2] Maude Abbott didn't graduate in medicine at McGill (she was too early for that) but by 1918 she was not only on the McGill staff, she had become one of the most famous members of the staff. She had become a world-famous figure, a scholar of impressive proportions, winning international acclaim for the university as well as for herself. She was a very solid reminder, right there on the McGill campus, that a woman could be scholarly and could be worth educating.

Maude Abbott had been born a scholar. She had a scholar's quick mind that could grasp the essentials of a problem, and she had a scholar's slow patience, the thoroughness that could keep her painstakingly working on a project for years on end. She was made for the academic world. Even as a child she was earnestly and very consciously seeking knowledge, reading everything she could lay her hands on — from *Little Women* to Macaulay — and keeping a diary in which, time and again, she wrote of her longing for a formal education. Although she was taught by a governess, and taught very thoroughly, her great wish was to go to school. It would be such *fun* to study with other girls. Think of the challenge! Think of the 'loveliness' of knowing that success would depend entirely on one's own efforts! And think of the joy of learning such exciting subjects as Latin and German!

Strange entries for a child's diary.

Maude had a happy childhood, in spite of her frustrations about schooling and in spite of the fact that she was, to all intents, an orphan. Her parents' marriage had been a failure and her father had left home before Maude was born. Then her mother had died while she was a small baby. Maude and her sister, Alice, had been taken in by their maternal grandparents, legally adopted by them, given their name of Abbott and brought up by them at St Andrews East, the small Scottish town in Quebec. Maude had been born at St Andrews in 1869 and she was to remain strongly attached to the town all her life. It had been a British garrison town and, in a way, it represented her dual heritage: an English-speaking community and yet part of French Canada. Maude was French Canadian on her father's side. Her real name was Maude Babin.

But she was brought up in an English-speaking environment and her education was to be in English: it was to Miss Symmers and Smith School in Montreal that she was sent when eventually her great wish was granted. That was a marvellous time for Maude. At last all the joy and 'loveliness' were hers. But she wasn't satisfied for long, for this was only a stepping-stone. No sooner was she settled in at school, happily mastering theorems and learning passages from Caesar than she developed a further ambition: to go on to university.

In Montreal at that time there was very little higher education of any type available to girls. There was only one high school and just a few private schools like the one Maude attended, but while these schools could coach the girls for their matriculation exams, the matric didn't qualify them for university. Or rather, it qualified them, but they weren't admitted, not even in Arts. It was the old problem: the objection to mixed classes. Separate classes were out of the question — they would be impossibly expensive — and co-education was held to be far too risky, even though the students would be studying such modest subjects as literature or language. But, of course, this was only an excuse. The real reason was that McGill had no desire to let women enter its all-male stronghold. It was unwilling, as much as unable, to finance separate classes.

However in 1884, while Maude was at Miss Symmers' school, the financial excuse was demolished. In that year, Donald Smith (later Lord Strathcona) offered McGill $50,000 for the higher education of women, a donation that he increased to $120,000 two years later. So McGill had little choice. Gracefully, if unhappily, it agreed to accept women in Arts and it established the Donalda Department for the handful of unnaturally ambitious women who had been begging to be admitted. This department had been in existence a full year by the time Maude Abbott matriculated from school in 1885.

Maude matriculated so brilliantly that she won a scholarship to McGill and this removed her own financial barriers. A university education was an expense that her family could ill afford, for her grandfather had died by this time, but since Maude had won the scholarship and had set her heart on going to McGill, Grandmother Abbott agreed to let her enrol. However, Maude was obliged to wait a year before she could really get started, because her grandmother was worried about a smallpox epidemic in Montreal; but in 1886 she was in the city, excitedly signing on at McGill as a First Year Arts student.

The four years that followed were probably four of the happiest years of Maude's life. 'I was literally in love with McGill,' she wrote.[3] She entered with zest into the student life, helping to form such organizations as the Delta Sigma Debating Society, and acting as the Donalda Editor of the *McGill Fortnightly,* thoroughly enjoying herself both in work and play, and making some lasting friendships. One of these was with a girl called Octavia Grace Ritchie.

Grace Ritchie (later Dr Ritchie-England) was two years ahead of Maude. She had been the dominant character in getting an Arts course for women started at McGill and she had been one of its original students. She was a very determined young woman, a courageous fighter and committed feminist, and she was to lead the way for Maude in medicine as well as in Arts. For Grace Ritchie intended to graduate in medicine. And she hoped to do so at McGill.

Grace had an excellent platform from which to launch her medical campaign. Literally a platform. She had been chosen as Class Valedictorian at her graduation ceremony — the girl who would make the speech on behalf of McGill's first women graduates — so here was an opportunity not to be missed: there would be a large audience and just the right audience. Grace worked carefully on her address, and on the day of her graduation she made a public appeal to McGill to continue its enlightened work, formally requesting the university to start a medical course for women.

It was a courageous attempt, but it didn't go down at all well. The Principal had censored the appeal when he had looked over the draft of Grace's speech and he was not pleased when she read it regardless.[4] Very few of the staff were pleased. Grace was accused of forwardness, of disobedience, of lack of decorum, of ungratefulness. She had been granted the extraordinary privilege of being allowed to study at McGill, she had just been honoured with a BA, and instead of saying 'thank you', here she was asking for more, asking to study medicine!

Grace departed from McGill in both a cloud of disgrace and a blaze of glory and she signed on as a student at the Kingston Women's Medical College. But she had launched the campaign and, by this time, Maude Abbott was just about ready to take it over from her. Maude had only recently decided on a medical career. It hadn't been a long-standing ambition. Her aim had simply been to do well at McGill, and she hadn't really considered what she would do afterwards, until one of her girlfriends suggested medicine. Medicine? Why not? It would be interesting and it would be challenging. And very worth while. The more Maude thought it through, the more suitable it seemed. Yes . . . she would become a physician. If her grandmother approved.

'May I be a doctor?' she asked her grandmother.

'Dear child, you may be anything you like,' Mrs Abbott replied.

This was very true. Maude Abbott could have been anything she liked. She had the brains and the determination, as well as family backing, and we can only be thankful that her friend suggested medicine. It is strange that some of our most outstanding women doctors slipped into medicine almost accidentally — because friends or husbands suggested it, because the family needed a doctor, or because a knowledge of the subject would be a useful accessory in the mission field. They weren't all Augusta Stowes, knowing from childhood that they wanted to be Mrs Doctor. Nor were they all feminists. The only real feminist campaign that Maude Abbott ever conducted was the one she took over from Grace Ritchie — the effort to get a medical course for women started at McGill — and the motivation behind that was love of McGill, the longing to stay on for another few years, rather than any very strong feelings about the rights of women.

Nevertheless the motivation was strong — Maude's beloved Mc-Gill just *had* to accept her as a medical student — and in 1889, before she had even graduated in Arts, Maude sent a letter to the Faculty of Medicine, humbly petitioning them to set up a course for women. She hinted at what they were missing: 'Already earnest students have been obliged to leave Montreal in order to seek a medical education in other (and inferior) universities.'[5] She suggested that the Principal was not opposed to the project. She begged for a speedy reply. And she remained Yours Respectfully.

The reply was very speedy. And short, and negative.

It was also predictable. Maude can hardly have been surprised and she doesn't seem to have been dismayed. She had probably expected that her letter would be no more than an opening skirmish, and she now gathered her friends and supporters — and her energies — to launch a full-scale attack. Suspecting that cost would again be the chief barrier (or at any rate the chief excuse) she started a fund-raising campaign and this took off so enthusiastically that by the end of the first week she and her friends had raised twelve thousand dollars. At this rate, it looked as if they would be able to establish a McGill Medical College for Women, not merely a separate course.

But their optimism was premature. In this instance, mere money was not to be the answer. In spite of the encouraging support, only a few members of the Faculty of Medicine spoke out in favour of the women, and their voices were hardly heard among the shouts which came from the opposition. Dr George Fenwick, the Professor of Surgery, was one of the most adamant. He was not the same Dr Fenwick who had given the Queen's women such a hard time, but his reactions were very similar: he threatened to resign if a medical course was started for women. And Dr Francis Wayland Campbell, Dean of Medicine of the University of Bishop's College, was even more dangerous: although he didn't mind the idea of educating women in medicine, he hit on the weak point — or what too many were delighted to consider the weak point: the failings of females.

'They may be useful in some departments in medicine,' he said, 'but in difficult work, in surgery, for instance, they would not have the nerve. And can you think of a patient in a critical case, waiting for half an hour while the medical lady fixes her bonnet or adjusts her bustle?'[6]

This witticism was produced in 1889 when Charlotte Whitehead Ross had been practising at Whitemouth for nearly a decade, coping with the most horrible emergencies without pausing to pretty herself first. Plenty of women had proved that they did have the nerve and weren't concerned with bustles and bonnets. Besides, the precedent had already been established. The universities of Victoria College, of Queen's, Trinity and Toronto were all granting medical degrees to women, and both Dalhousie and Manitoba were willing to do so, though at this date they hadn't yet enrolled any women medics. Even more startling — though Dr Campbell may not have known of it — was that Dr Elizabeth Simpson Mitchell, a graduate of Queen's, had recently set up a practice right in Montreal and had actually been licensed by the College of Physicians and Surgeons.

So, in a way, these men were fighting a battle that had already been lost. But McGill's Faculty of Medicine hadn't lost its battle, its own private battle against a monstrous regiment of medical females. Let other universities lower their standards if they wanted to, but McGill would stand firm.

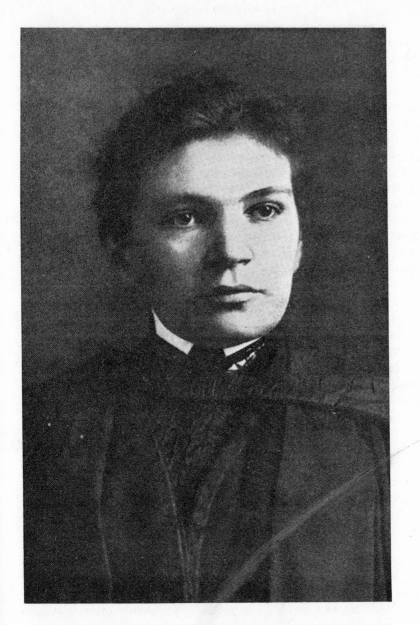

Dr Maude Abbott at the time of her graduation, 1894

This was a great blow to Maude. And it wasn't really eased when the Medical Faculty of the University of Bishop's College offered to take her on as a student. Bishop's Medical College was in Montreal,[7] a rival to McGill's Faculty of Medicine, and Maude certainly listed it among the 'inferior' universities that she had mentioned in her letter. Even so, she accepted. At least she would remain in Montreal. Besides, some of the hospital instruction would be given by McGill professors — there would be a tenuous connection with her beloved Alma Mater.

It was partly because of the hospital instruction that Bishop's had decided to take this step. Grace Ritchie had been doing clinical work at the Montreal Western Hospital during her summer vacations from Kingston, and the Bishop's staff had come to know and respect her. When they heard that she had been granted a ticket to walk the wards at the Montreal General, they offered to take her on as a third year student. They liked Grace, and they felt it would be easier for her to do all her training in Montreal. And, of course, it would also put them one up on McGill.

If Bishop's was going to admit one woman, why not admit two or three? The university wrote around, issuing invitations. This was most promising, but unfortunately it didn't represent a breakthrough. Only twelve women ever graduated from Bishop's medical faculty — not because of any disturbance within the university, but because of the opposition of the Montreal hospitals.

All universities naturally had to be able to offer hospital facilities to their medical students. One of the advertised Advantages of the Woman's Medical College in Toronto was that it could offer its young ladies access to the Toronto hospitals where special arrangements had been made for them, such as seats in the operating theatre and bedside instruction in the wards. But special arrangements, or even the admission of women, was not so popular in Montreal and it wasn't long before the hospitals were refusing to give women students tickets of admission.

This was also partly Grace Ritchie's doing. Her ticket of admission — such a novelty — had been followed by applications from a number of her fellow students at Kingston, who also wanted to walk the wards during their summer vacation. The hospitals panicked. Had they set a precedent? Was Miss Ritchie the thin end of the wedge? Was there going to be a great invasion of women students? Grace wrote frantically to Maude, telling her that tickets were being refused to women and that she should send in her twenty-dollar fee immediately. Maude sent her fee to the hospital, but even so, her ticket was witheld.

She was now in an impossible situation. She had already started to attend classes at Bishop's but unless she had access to a Montreal hospital she wouldn't be able to complete her course there. Hospital experience was a mandatory part of the course. Maude began to inquire about other universities — was the Woman's Medical College of Pennsylvania superior? — but while she was doing so, her predicament became public. Maude was in such an absurd dilemma and one that was so blatantly unfair that she naturally aroused public sympathy, and the battle was fought for her (largely by people she didn't even know) while she sat at home in St Andrews, reading booklets about Pennsylvania, trying not to read the newspapers — it was so alarming to see her name in them — and worrying about the storm she had inadvertently caused, worrying that people would think her forward and immodest and that the controversy would harm both her reputation and her career.

It did neither. In the midst of all the publicity, the hospital ticket arrived quietly by post.

Having survived two campaigns, and finally been accepted both by university and hospital, Maude should have been feeling triumphant at this time. She was well on the road to becoming a physician and she had the honour of being in the first group of women medical students accepted by Bishop's. She should have been on top of the world. But the whole thing was a let-down, mainly because she was at Bishop's not McGill. It was all dreary and drab. And, of course, inferior.

She didn't even like her fellow students. She found them rough and with 'low standards' compared to the McGill boys, and in their turn, the students didn't like her. They thought her a 'swot'. She was too eager to learn, too high in her marks and too forward, pushing herself to the front of the class so that she could see what was being demonstrated. Maude must have made it obvious that she was at Bishop's only for the education, and this too may have caused resentment. So may her attitude to her fellow students. They might have forgiven her her eagerness and her brilliant marks if she had flirted a little. But Maude had neither the nature nor desire to act the coquette, not with the Bishop's boys at any rate.

Consequently she was lonely at Bishop's and she was miserable, and her grandmother's death at this time added to her misery and loneliness. Often she was the only woman in the class: Grace Ritchie graduated in 1891 and the other girl, Mary Fyffe, didn't attend the third and fourth year clinics. However, neither Maude's private loneliness nor her personal tragedy affected her academic performance. In 1894 she graduated brilliantly, winning the Senior Anatomy Prize as well as the Chancellor's Prize for the best examination. Maude had won the Lord Stanley Gold Medal when she had graduated in Arts in 1890, so she was very clearly justifying the education of women. Already she was far more accomplished than most of her classmates but, even so, she didn't feel that her education was complete. There was plenty more to learn, plenty more which *should* be learnt — so she and her sister set off for Vienna, Maude to study medicine and Alice to study music.

Vienna was the Mecca of the medical world, the shrine of all wisdom, and anyone who was seriously in search of knowledge just had to worship there for a few years. Maude was to spend three years in Europe, three wonderful years, first in Zurich, then in Vienna and then in Britain. In both Zurich and Vienna the universities admitted women, and Maude seems to have taken just about every course that was open to her — including pathology, which was later to become one of her specialties. In Britain, she concentrated more on practical work, interning in a women's hospital in Glasgow and working as clinical assistant at an asylum in Birmingham. And then, in 1897, finally considering herself qualified to open a small practice for women and children, she returned to Montreal.

It was inevitable that Maude would open a practice for women and children. There was no real alternative if she wanted to work in Montreal. She had no particular desire to spend her life delivering babies and diagnosing whooping-cough — it wasn't challenging enough — but it looked as if it would be her lot. It was the lot of most medical women. In spite of her brilliant academic performance and in spite of the fact that she had spent eleven years studying and training, she was faced with the prospect of running an ordinary practice, ministering to the needs of ordinary patients, just like any ordinary graduate who had had to struggle to pass his finals. A life sentence. The future looked very grey.

In addition, her sister was ill. Alice had contracted diphtheria while she was in Vienna and this had been followed by a breakdown which had affected her mind. She was to remain an invalid for life and Maude was just beginning to realize this. Maude never fully accepted that her sister was incurable, but already in 1897 she must have known that her own strength and her own earnings were going to have to support them both from now on. So she was not a happy young woman, nor an optimistic one, when only a few weeks after establishing her practice, she took a walk through McGill campus.

It cannot have been chance that took Maude Abbott into McGill: the chances are that she couldn't keep away. And it wasn't really chance that she met Dr Charles Martin, her former supervisor at the Montreal General and the future Dean of Medicine at McGill. Maude was sure to have met Dr Martin sooner or later: they moved in the same worlds. Nor was it chance that Maude began to talk about the slides of pigmentation of cirrhosis which she had made in Vienna: she was absorbingly interested in them. And, finally, Dr Martin's reaction wasn't a chance response. Long ago he had recognized Maude's potential, and that day in the McGill campus he also recognized her misery.

The upshot of this almost predictable meeting was that Dr Martin set Maude to work on a study of functional heart murmurs, and arranged for her to show her cirrhosis slides to Dr John Adami, who was Pathologist at the Royal Victoria Hospital and Professor of Pathology at McGill. Dr Adami was extremely interested and he too set Maude to work — on a piece of pathological research connected with the slides. Maude continued with her practice, but she had her foot in the door and that door was to open very quickly when the paper she wrote for Dr Martin was read for her at the Medico-Chirurgical Society (she couldn't present it herself, for women were not admitted). While the members were praising the paper, Dr Adami, who was present at the meeting, proposed that women should be admitted to the society and that Dr Maude Abbott should be nominated for membership. Carried without a quibble — though a motion to admit women had been turned down the previous year. The paper Maude wrote for Professor Adami was equally successful. It was a very thorough piece of research, which took her two years to complete, but in 1900 it was presented for her at the Pathological Society of London — the first time a research paper by a woman had ever been given there.

At last Maude Abbott was well on her way, taking her place in the world of men. She hadn't fought her way in, she hadn't charmed her way in. She hadn't even contrived it. But there she was, tentatively but very solidly inside the locked gates. The impressive thing about Dr Maude Abbott was that she was admitted to this world purely on her abilities — not as a woman, but as a scholar. Her work was of such a high standard that nobody could afford to ignore it.

For this reason the gates of McGill were also reopened to her, in spite of her sex. In 1898 she was appointed Assistant Curator of the university's medical museum and the following year she was promoted to the position of Curator. This seems a most unlikely appointment — unlikely from McGill's point of view — until one realizes that Professor Adami may have had a hand in it. He had already recognized Maude's abilities, and as head of McGill's Pathological Department, he was Director of the museum. It was almost certainly his influence which got Maude this most suitable position. And it was extremely suitable. It was not only within Maude's beloved McGill, but it provided just the type of work she was most fitted for.

The job that Curator Abbott was required to do was to set the museum in order. There was a wealth of material here, but it was in such a muddle that it was virtually useless as a teaching aid. The pathological section particularly needed attention. Specimens had been collected ever since the medical college started — there were hundreds of them, in bottles and jars, on this shelf, under that bench — and none of them had been catalogued or classified. Here was a task worthy of Maude's abilities. For the museum didn't merely need an organizer: it needed a lover, someone who could devote years to its care, someone with the knowledge and intelligence to understand the specimens, someone with the thoroughness to trace their histories, someone who would fondly nurture the collection and develop it into a museum worthy of McGill. Maude took on the job with eagerness, an eagerness that never flagged. When, years later, her catalogue of the collection was finally printed, it proved to be far more than a catalogue: it had become a detailed textbook on gross pathology.

Before Maude started her classification of the museum specimens, she was sent to the United States to study other museums. At Johns Hopkins in Baltimore she met Sir William Osler, the brilliant Canadian physician and medical historian who was one of the most famous teachers of medicine in his day. Since Dr Osler had supplied many of the museum specimens during his years in Montreal, he was greatly interested in the project and he was to act powerfully as its absent friend — and as Maude's too. '[His] keen interest in my work,' she wrote, 'and broad human sympathy pierced the veil of my youthful shyness with a personal stimulus that aroused my intellect to its most passionate endeavour.'[8]

There is no doubt that Sir William Osler did stimulate Maude's work, but she had never lacked passionate endeavour. And her youthful shyness does not seem to have been so very shy at this time. Hearing about her work at the museum, the students had taken to dropping in there to chat with Dr Abbott and to learn about the specimens she was classifying. They were drawn to her as much as to the museum: her enthusiasm was magnetic. However busy she was, she could always take the time to explain and discuss — and before long all the final year students were coming in groups to be given demonstrations on the museum specimens. These demonstrations became so popular that in 1904 they were placed on the curriculum as a compulsory part of the course.

Maude was now extremely busy, happily busy, on a number of different projects: she still kept up her private practice, she was Curator of McGill's Medical Museum, Demonstrator at the university, and she was also at work on a number of research projects. And this was only the beginning. Throughout her career she was continually taking on new jobs, without any thought of dropping those she had already started. In 1907 she organized the International Association of Medical Museums — a mammoth task — and she became its permanent international secretary *and* brought out its Bulletin. In the meantime she was doing a great deal of research on congenital heart disease, writing histories and research papers, attending meetings of scientific and medical societies . . . and all with total concentration.

Quite apart from the high calibre of her work, the very size of it is staggering. Her bibliography lists more than one hundred publications and many of them were scientific papers based on detailed research. Others were histories — histories of vaccination, of nursing, of St Andrews and, of course, of McGill — and these also required considerable research. Some were huge tomes, like the Osler Memorial volume which included articles from just about everyone who had known Sir William and which took seven years to complete. Others were simply chapters for books on medicine, but they weren't at all simple. They, too, were given her most passionate endeavour. Dr Abbott couldn't do anything half-heartedly.

One work which increased her prestige enormously was the section she wrote on congenital heart disease for Sir William Osler's *System of Medicine*. It was prestige enough to be one of the authors, but Sir William knew what he was doing when he asked Maude to contribute. He had to wait two years for her section to come in, which wasn't excessive considering the work involved, and when it did arrive, his judgement was more than justified. He was absolutely delighted.

I knew you would write a good article but I did not expect one of such extraordinary merit. It is by far and away the very best thing ever written on the subject in English — possibly in any language. I cannot begin to tell you how much I appreciate the care and trouble you have taken. . . . For years it will be the standard work on the subject. . . .[9]

There were many who shared Dr Osler's opinion. By 1908, when her monograph for the *System of Medicine* was published, Dr. Abbott had gathered a large following of admirers. But her reputation was greater in other countries than it was at home. At McGill, most people thought of her, rather tolerantly, as a form of female absented-minded-professor, a 'character' who worked in a mess — papers everywhere — who dropped handkerchiefs and notebooks as she walked along, who never could find her train ticket and who, in the stress of the moment, might appear with her skirt on back-to-front or her hair all blown about. She was the soul of kindness, nobody could deny that, but she was considered an amusing character rather than a celebrity. Of course such people as Dr Adami and Sir William Osler recognized her outstanding qualities, and they had done so from the first, but on the whole McGill didn't realize what a very remarkable figure it had in its midst.

The realization came gradually, but by 1910 McGill had to sit up and take notice. Dr Abbott had become such a famous international figure by then that she could no longer be overlooked, and at last the Alma Mater acted. It awarded Dr Abbott an honorary MD CM and appointed her Lecturer in Pathology.

The honorary degree must have brought Maude a great deal of pleasure. To have a medical degree from McGill, from *her* McGill, was a wonderful accolade. So, too, was the lectureship. It wasn't a sideline thing like the post of Curator. She was now in the mainstream of the teaching staff.

Both the honorary degree and the lectureship placed McGill in a very strange position. The university was still refusing to give women medical education, yet it had granted a woman a Doctorate in Medicine and appointed her to the staff. However, McGill doesn't seem to have found this inconsistent. Or uncomfortable. Nor did Dr Abbott's unquestionable brilliance tempt the university to venture farther in the direction of female education. It wasn't for another eight years that young ladies were admitted to McGill's Faculty of Medicine, and even then the admission was very cautious.

In 1917, four of McGill's female Arts graduates were allowed to take first year medicine, provided they registered for the B sc rather than the MD degree (there seems to have been some hope that they might be persuaded to finish their course in Toronto). But the performance of these four young women was too exceptional to ignore. One of them, Jessie Boyd, headed the lists of her entire year; two of the others had aggregate honours in all subjects, and the fourth wasn't lagging far behind — she came thirteenth in a class of seventy-two.[10] McGill could hardly hold out against such results, not in the twentieth century, and in the following session the four women were formally admitted to the Faculty of Medicine. A fifth woman, Winifred Blampin, who had done her first year in Toronto,[11] was also admitted. All five graduated in 1922.

At last women could study medicine at McGill — but not on an equal footing with men. The university was still being cautious. Before young ladies could take up the study of medicine, they were required either to have obtained a BA or a B sc or to have done two years in Arts at McGill 'and thus give evidence that they are sufficiently mature and otherwise qualified to take up the study of the professional branches.'[12] Men were required to give no such evidence of maturity.

Even so, it was a breakthrough, and it was hailed as such by the *Canadian Medical Association Journal*. The CMAJ gave women's 'splendid work towards winning the war' as the reason for McGill's change of policy, but it is very likely that Maude Abbott herself was just as powerful a reason. Her work had been so outstanding that it must have influenced the university. Probably the only reason why the *Journal's* editorial didn't mention this, was that it was almost certainly Maude Abbott herself who wrote the editorial.

Dr Abbott had taken over as Editor of the CMAJ during the war, and she was to remain on the editorial board for the rest of her life. She was still collecting new jobs, and she continued to do so. Her next project — another huge task — was the cataloguing of the Canadian Army Medical Museum, to which she was appointed Acting Curator. And then, in 1921, she took on yet another job, becoming Lecturer on the History of Nursing at the McGill School of Graduate Nurses.

She was to gain several lectureships and professorships before the end of her career. For two years she held the post of Professor of Pathology and Bacteriology at the Woman's Medical College of Pennsylvania, and in 1925 she was made Assistant Professor of Medical Research at McGill, a position she held until her retirement. Dr Abbott could have been professor at other universities too — she received several offers — but she couldn't bring herself to leave McGill. She was only tempted to Philadelphia for a few years because the college offered her double salary when she refused. Maude wasn't a rich woman — much of her work brought no salary at all — and she constantly needed money for her sister's care. So she agreed to go to Philadelphia, but only for a limited period and clearly on the understanding that she was on loan from McGill. She wouldn't leave McGill permanently.

But she had to do so when she reached retirement age. There was no appeal. In 1936, at the age of sixty-seven, Dr Maude Abbott sadly bade farewell to her Alma Mater. Yet although it was a sad farewell, it was a proud one, for McGill honoured Dr Abbott with an LLD which was formally bestowed on her at Convocation.

And so she retired from McGill, but of course she didn't stop working. Like so many women doctors, mere age wasn't going to remove Dr Abbott from her profession. She immediately set off on a lecture tour, busy as ever, and when she died in 1940, she had just embarked on a major work, a textbook on congenital heart disease which was to include an analysis of one thousand cases. An amazing undertaking for a seventy year old. She had even received a Carnegie Grant for the project.

The news of Maude Abbott's death was received with very real sorrow by members of the medical profession throughout the world. A personal friend had died as well as a most outstanding medical woman, and the many tributes contained as much warmth as admiration. It was typical that Dr Paul White of the New England Heart Association recalled her generosity, her kindheartedness, and her delightful enthusiasm, before moving on to make the impressive statement that ranked her among the giants of her profession: 'It is not simply as the world's authority on congenital heart disease that Maude Abbott will be best remembered, but as a living force in the medicine of her generation.'[13]

Even today, Maude Abbott continues to be a force in medicine, for two scholarships were given in her honour. One was instituted anonymously shortly before her death and the other, the Maude Abbott Scholarship Loan Fund, was established in her memory by the Federation of Medical Women of Canada. Dr Abbott had been one of the founders of the Federation in 1924, but she was really singled out for this distinction because of her unparalleled contribution as a medical *woman.*

More than anyone else, Dr Abbott had caused women to become accepted by the profession. She had shown the whole world just how much a woman doctor could achieve. She had been a signpost pointing the way: onwards, upwards and into — into all-male spheres of medicine. She may not have thought of herself as a pioneer or as an active suffragette, yet the very stature of her work pioneered for her, promoting the cause of women as effectively as if she had spent most of her life campaigning for equal rights. Her importance lies in the fact that she was accepted by men as a fellow-researcher, fellow-scholar, fellow-specialist. For Maude Abbott achieved equality with men, not by legislation, but by performance.

FIVE MONTREALERS

OCTAVIA GRACE RITCHIE-ENGLAND (Bishop's, 1891)

The first woman to graduate in medicine (and in Arts) in the Province of Quebec, Grace Ritchie completed her education by taking a course in Vienna. On her return to Canada, she married Dr Frank England and opened a general practice in Montreal.

Welfare work and women's suffrage were Dr Ritchie-England's two greatest concerns. She did a great deal for the Montreal poor, and in 1914 she was chosen as one of the women to represent Canada at the meeting in Rome of the International Council of Women. For many years she was Assistant Gynaecologist at Montreal's Western Hospital, and in 1930 she was chosen by the Liberal Party as their Federal candidate for Mount Royal. She died in Montreal in 1948, at the age of 80.

REGINA LEWIS-LANDAU (Bishop's, 1895)

Dr Lewis-Landau practised for some years in Montreal. She too was a suffragette, and she helped to organize the Jewish Young Ladies' Literary Society.

ELIZABETH SIMPSON MITCHELL (Queen's, 1888)

Elizabeth Mitchell was one of the Montrealers who studied medicine at the Women's Medical College in Kingston. Since she graduated outside the Province of Quebec, Dr Mitchell had difficulty in obtaining a licence to practise there, so she went to England and obtained the degree of MRCS Lond., which qualified her to practise in all British colonies and dominions. On her return to Montreal, she was therefore granted a licence (in 1889). Her name is the first woman's name to appear in the Register of the College of Physicians and Surgeons of Quebec. Dr Mitchell practised in Montreal until her retirement in 1908, when she went to England to look after her elderly parents. She died at Nashua, New Haven, in 1912.

MINNIE GOMERY (Bishop's, 1898)

Born in Birmingham, England, in 1875, Minnie Gomery was brought to Canada as a child. Her family settled at Huntingdon, P.Q. but they moved to Montreal a few years before Minnie enrolled at Bishop's. Since she couldn't get an internship in Montreal, Dr Gomery went to England after her graduation and there she trained in theology as well as medicine, in preparation for missionary work. She signed on with the Church Missionary Society who sent her to Kashmir, and she worked as an Anglican medical missionary until she retired in 1953 at the age of 78. She returned to Montreal and died there in 1967.

MARY RUNNELLS BIRD (Bishop's, 1900)
Mary Runnells (Mrs Bird) was born in Milton, P.Q. and after graduating from Bishop's she set up a practice in Montreal. However, her marriage to an Englishman — Charles Bird — took her overseas and she was in England when the First War broke out. She immediately volunteered for service and was appointed house surgeon at Eggington Hall Hospital in England. In 1922 Dr Bird and her husband returned to Montreal and she was given a staff position at the Montreal General Hospital and at the Child Welfare Clinic. She was 91 when she died.

McGILL'S FIRST WOMEN MEDICAL GRADUATES

JESSIE BOYD SCRIVER (McGill, 1922)

Jessie Boyd (Mrs Scriver) was born and educated in Montreal. On her graduation from McGill, she won the Wood Gold Medal for clinical medicine, and after interning in Montreal, she did postgraduate work in Boston for two years. Returning to Canada, she was appointed to the staff of the Royal Victoria Hospital, where she rose to become Head of Paediatrics. She was also a paediatrician at the Montreal Children's Hospital and a member of the staff of McGill University, where she became Professor of Paediatrics. Dr Scriver was President of the Canadian Paediatric Society, President of the Child Health Association of Montreal and, in 1939-40, President of the Federation of Medical Women of Canada. Dr Scriver has now retired from the practice of medicine, but she is still working. As the Archivist at the Montreal Children's Hospital, she is assembling a history of the hospital.

MARY CHILDS (McGill, 1922)

After her graduation, Dr Childs interned at the Montreal General Hospital. Paediatrics was also her specialty and she was very active in child welfare work throughout her career.

WINIFRED BLAMPIN (McGill, 1922)

In 1923, when Dr Maude Abbott was appointed to the Chair of Pathology at the Woman's Medical College of Pennsylvania, she took three women with her as her teaching staff. One of these was Winifred Blampin who was appointed Teaching Fellow in Pathology at the Woman's Medical College. Later Dr Blampin moved to California, where she specialized in allergies.

ELEANOR PERCIVAL (McGill, 1922)

Born and educated in Montreal, Eleanor Percival specialized in obstetrics and gynaecology and became a senior member of the staff of the Montreal General Hospital. She was also on the staff of the Royal Victoria Hospital and the Catherine Booth Hospital and she was Consulting Gynaecologist to the Reddy Memorial Hospital. For thirty years she was a member of the teaching staff of McGill University, rising to the position of Assistant Professor of Obstetrics and Gynaecology.

LILIAN IRWIN McDONALD (McGill, 1922)

Lilian Irwin (Mrs McDonald) specialized in anaesthesiology. After her marriage she moved from Montreal to Sault Ste Marie and she was still working as an anaesthetist when she died.

9

Peace and war

ONE OF THE difficulties that the women doctors had faced all along was that they hadn't been given the opportunity to prove themselves by performance, not in the 'masculine' areas of medicine. How could a woman prove herself a brilliant surgeon, if she wasn't given the chance either to train or practise in surgery? How could she become a radiologist if she wasn't allowed near an X-ray machine?

By the beginning of the twentieth century, Canadian women had certainly advanced a long way — they could study medicine now without too much opposition, and they could qualify and practise as doctors — but almost invariably they were restricted to female roles. If a woman specialized, then it would have to be in obstetrics or gynaecology. If she went into public health, it would be as an inspector of schoolchildren or as a child welfare officer. If she wanted to teach and to do so in Canada, it would have to be at the Ontario Medical College for Women. Women doctors were expected to do women's work. Even the missionaries generally found themselves opening hospitals for women, since that was the great need in the east. And although pioneering women like Charlotte Ross might be able to treat males as often as females, or act as surgeon as well as physician, such women were very rare. And Maude Abbott was unique.

Of course, one of the reasons for the female directioning of women doctors was that there was a very real need for women *as women* in medicine. Great attention was still being given to 'a woman's tender touch' (so much more suitable with children) and also to modesty. So there was a very necessary role for women to fill. But the reason why they were confined to this role was that they didn't have much choice. A great many branches of medicine were closed to them, simply because they couldn't get into the hospitals.

When Pearl Chute had interned at St Michael's in 1895, she was very likely the only woman intern in any hospital in Canada, and in any case it was an irregular affair, lasting only a few months. But times were changing and around the turn of the century a few women did begin to get taken on, such as Helen MacMurchy, who had interned at the Toronto General Hospital. Cautiously, some of the other hospitals followed suit, but women were the exception rather than the rule, and they were seldom real residents. Because of accommodation problems they didn't live in the hospital (they couldn't possibly lodge with the men!). Nor did they necessarily get an appointment after their internship.

It was partly to remedy this situation that the Women's College Hospital was founded in Toronto. If there was a hospital staffed entirely by women, then women would not only be able to get hospital training, they would be able to try their hands at specialized work. However, the Women's College Hospital didn't suddenly spring into being in response to a loud demand for opportunity. It developed gradually from the Dispensary attached to the Ontario Medical College for Women.[1]

The Dispensary had been started in a very modest manner in 1896, holding clinics in two rooms in Sackville Street, but in 1898 it had been given space in the basement of the Ontario Medical College for Women, and clinics were held there as an adjunct to the College. A young American girl, Anna McFee, was its founding spirit; she was still a student at the college in 1896, but she had seen similar women's college clinics in the States and felt they could usefully be held in Toronto too. Having made her contribution to Canadian medicine, she returned home to New York. But she had got the Women's Dispensary started, and it was to treat more than twenty-five thousand patients before the Ontario Medical College for Women closed in 1906.[2]

With the closing of the college, the Dispensary became an institution in its own right. It moved house, took most of the staff of the medical college with it, and grew in size and reputation until in 1915 it became a fully-fledged hospital in a building on Rusholme Road. Of course, the facilities were fairly limited at first (the hospital didn't move to its ten-storey building on Grenville Street until 1935) but already by 1918 it had built on a new wing and was ordering X-ray machinery and building a pathology department. Women doctors at last had a hospital in Canada where they could train and specialize in non-female branches of medicine. At last they had a setting in which they could prove themselves by their performance.

They had also had another opportunity to do so by this time, a very challenging opportunity and one that was far more widely publicized: the First World War. 'Male man' might be able to over-look — or even scoff at — the work being performed in a women's hospital, but no man would feel like joking about women doctors who were up there at the Front, extracting bullets, amputating legs, valiantly saving lives, and quietly doing their duty without a mur-mur while bombs and shells fell around them. Such gallantry couldn't be overlooked, especially by those who had witnessed it. Neither could the work of the women who stayed at home, filling in for men who went off to the war, taking over their jobs and perform-ing them perfectly competently. The war not only gave women a chance to act. It gave their actions the chance to be noticed.

By 1918 a great many of our women doctors had therefore gained wide praise for their work. Some had gained their reputations in hospitals in Canada, others had done so in field hospitals in France or Serbia, and some had done both. Irma LeVasseur did both. She was the young Quebecoise who was still at school when Mme Bruère was opening her practice in Montreal, but Dr LeVasseur was in her thirties when the war broke out, and already she was making a name for herself in Quebec.[3]

Irma LeVasseur has often been acclaimed as the first woman ever to practise medicine in the Province of Quebec, and although this isn't true, she was probably the first French-Canadian woman to do so. Elizabeth Walker Bruère had little, if any, French blood. Such people as Charlotte Ross and Grace Ritchie-England were decidedly Anglo-Saxon, and although Maude Abbott (Babin) was partly of

French extraction, she worked within an English environment. But Irma LeVasseur was entirely and thoroughly French Canadian.

She had been born in Quebec City in 1878, the daughter of the journalist Louis-Nazaire LeVasseur and she had been brought up in French surroundings, sent to the Couvent de Jésus-Marie at the age of nine, and educated there until she was sixteen years old. When Irma left the convent in 1894, she had already decided on a career in medicine but, of course, her problem was where to study. Neither Laval nor the Université de Montréal accepted women, nor did McGill, and the situation at Bishop's was so uncertain (because of the hospital stand against women) that it was hardly worth trying for entrance there.

Irma had learnt English, so language was no barrier, but she didn't choose one of Canada's English-speaking colleges. She signed on at the Minnesota University College of Medicine at St Paul in the United States,[4] probably because of the French connection with the city. It had been settled by the French and by refugees from the Red River Colony, and in the late 1890's there were about a thousand French Canadians living there. Although they were only a small minority, at least it was a link with home.

Irma graduated in 1900 and she then stayed on in the States, setting up a practice in New York. For a time it looked as if she might become one of the increasing number of Canadian women graduates who were establishing themselves in the States because of the greater scope there. But, fortunately for the children of Quebec, she decided to make her career in her own country, and she returned to Canada after two years of general practice.

When she returned home, Dr LeVasseur discovered that she would need a special licence if she was to practise in Quebec — not because she was a woman, but because her degree was from Minnesota. This proved to be more of a formality than a problem, and in 1903 a private bill was passed in the Legislative Assembly,[5] officially allowing her to be registered with the College of Physicians and Surgeons. Fully qualified, and officially accepted as a doctor, she began to practise in Montreal, but this didn't last any longer than her New York practice. Dr LeVasseur found herself becoming increasingly interested in the health of young children and, in 1905, she set off for Paris to take a course in paediatrics. It was only after she had done a postgraduate course in France and had worked in hospitals for sick children there and in Germany that she returned to Canada and really began what was to be her life's work.

The work for which Dr LeVasseur was to become famous was paediatrics. This was a new and relatively untried branch of medicine, not previously considered a specialist subject, and in Quebec virtually nothing had been done in this area until Dr LeVasseur started practising. At the time there was no hospital which specialized in the treatment of young children and there was a very real need for such a hospital. The infant mortality rate was exceptionally high, and there were thousands of poor children from crowded homes, born weak and suffering from generations of malnutrition, who had little chance of survival when they became ill. They sickened at home and died at home, and it was almost taken for granted that they should do so.

This situation changed in 1907, thanks to the concern of Dr LeVasseur. Fresh from her studies in Europe, she arrived back home in a campaigning mood, ready to heal and nurse the children of Quebec. Naturally her first task was to form a hospital where they could be treated, and she enlisted the help of Madame Louis de Gaspé Beaubien and Madame Alfred Thibaudeau, two society women who were well known for their charity work; with their backing and support, she founded the Hôpital Ste-Justine in Montreal, a hospital which was to cater specifically to patients under the age of two. Dr LeVasseur ran the hospital and Madame de Gaspé Beaubien became its president.

Madame de Gaspé Beaubien has often been credited with all the honour for founding the hospital, and certainly Dr LeVasseur couldn't have done it without her support, but Madame de Gaspé Beaubien never had any doubts herself about who was the driving force and just how significant that force was. Speaking of Dr LeVasseur later in life, she said: 'Elle fut l'instigatrice de notre hôpital et par conséquent, fut au point de départ de la pédiatrie dans notre province. Je remercie Dieu de m'avoir placée sur la route de cette femme remarquable.'[6]

Having been at the *point de départ* of paediatric work in the province, in fact having taken on the role of Quebec's pioneering paediatrician, this *femme remarquable* didn't stop there. Later in her life she was to found yet another children's hospital, this time with the co-operation of Dr René Fortier and Dr Edouard Samson.

Backed by a ladies committee, they established a small hospital in Quebec City in 1923. This was the Hêpital de l'Enfant-Jésus, which is now one of the largest and busiest hospitals in the city.

Irma LeVasseur served on the staff of l'Hôpital de l'Enfant-Jésus, as she had at the Hôpital Ste-Justine, but in 1927 she set up her own paediatric clinic and this was to be the centre for her work. By the time she died in 1964, she was one of the best known paediatricians in the province of Quebec, with an outstanding career behind her — and also a degree from Laval. Laval had awarded her an honorary degree in 1950 to mark the fiftieth anniversary of her graduation from Minnesota. Fifty glorious years — but there were other years of glory too. Besides gaining fame for her work in paediatrics, Dr LeVasseur had also gained fame as a First War heroine.

She had volunteered for service early in the war, in April, 1915, and she had embarked for Europe in a team with four male doctors. Their destination was Serbia, where doctors were urgently required — to help the sick rather than the wounded, for the country was being ravaged by a typhus epidemic, which was to kill more than 300,000 people before it had run its course.[7] Typhus had entered Serbia with the invading Austrian army, and although the Austrians had been beaten back beyond the frontiers, the disease they had brought with them remained, claiming far more victims than the actual fighting. Almost every town needed medical aid, and when the Quebec team arrived they therefore split up, Irma being sent to Kraguyevats in central Serbia.

She immediately set to work immunizing the population of the city, at the rate of a thousand a day. She organized a hospital, requisitioned four Austrian prisoners to help her, and started to isolate the diseased from the wounded. All her formidable energies were channelled into the work of at least containing the disease. But it was an impossible task. There weren't enough medical supplies or medical personnel, and there were far too many sick — so many that there were no beds for most of them and they were laid on the floor, or on bundles of straw, the dead often lying beside the living. They lay there in rows and they died there in rows, and were buried by the hundred in huge ditches which were covered over with quicklime.

Meanwhile Dr LeVasseur was working day and night — and she was working under constant enemy bombardment. Although the

Austrians had initially been driven back, the German invasion which began in 1915 was more successful, and before long, Dr Le-Vasseur was obliged to withdraw her unit from Kraguyevats to avoid capture. She set up another hospital in a barracks at Gorni Milanovats, only thirty miles back, now taking in almost as many wounded as diseased, and still being overwhelmed by the numbers of those who needed medical attention. Here conditions were even worse than they had been in Kraguyevats. There was hardly any food — black bread and goatmeat was about all that was available — and sometimes the doctor had to kill the goats herself. It wasn't nice but it was necessary, for the boiled goatmeat made a nourishing bouillon for the sick. Even so, it wasn't enough on its own, and there was virtually nothing else. There was no flour, no sugar, no milk — and there came a time when there weren't any medicines either.

Dr LeVasseur found herself faced with a desperate situation where she could do little for her patients except isolate those with typhus, provide the living with bouillon, and see that ditches were dug for the dead. She was both frustrated and exhausted, and yet she kept on smiling bravely, silently encouraging both patients and staff (silently, because she couldn't speak a word of the language!).

This should have been her darkest hour, but worse was yet to come for the whole of Serbia was to fall before the enemy. As the enemy advanced, the hospitals had to retreat with their patients. Like other allied hospital units, like foreign diplomats and Serbian soldiers, like thousands of near-starving men, women and children, Irma LeVasseur took part in the Great Retreat, moving back and farther back before the advancing enemy, walking much of the way, struggling by foot over the Albanian mountains towards escape through the ports of the Adriatic Sea. More than 700,000 people are said to have died on this terrible journey, but Irma LeVasseur, that tough and determined Quebecoise, made it to the coast. She survived this terrible ordeal to return to Canada — and, eventually, to resume her career in paediatrics.

It would be hard to say whether Dr LeVasseur deserves the greater glory for her work among the dying in Serbia or among the newly born in Quebec, but one thing is certain. By her performance in both peace and war, she added enormously to the prestige of women doctors. While it was an individual contribution rightly bringing her personally both fame and acclaim, the reputation of all medical women was increased because of her performance.

Every woman who served in the war brought credit to her profession as well as to herself, and a great many did serve in the war, though not all as actively as Dr LeVasseur. Many served in England, for their work was needed in the hospitals there, in convalescent hospitals, base hospitals, and even in general hospitals which had little connection with the war. By working in them, women could release a male doctor for active duty. Understandably, the Front wasn't considered at all suitable for women. Nevertheless, a good number of them saw active service: another of our women doctors in Serbia was Dr Ella Scarlett Synge of Vancouver. She set out in 1915 as commander of the Vancouver Women's Volunteer Reserve and she and her nurses established themselves in the district of Batochina.[8] But she too was forced to retire before the enemy advance. Other women saw active service in France and Belgium, in just about every theatre of war. Singly and in groups, working under one ally or another, they managed to get themselves into the thick of the fighting.

How they did so depended largely on their own initiative, for at the beginning of the war they couldn't simply join up: there was no women's army until 1917 when the Women's Army Auxiliary Force was formed, and of course there was no place for women in the regular army. Irma LeVasseur had volunteered with a group of Quebec men, Ella Scarlett Synge had formed and led her own group of Vancouver nurses and that was generally how it was done. If a woman wanted to serve overseas, then she either joined or formed a hospital unit, and these units then offered their services to the Red Cross or to one of the allied governments, and were sent wherever they were most needed.

One of the most famous of the women's units was the Scottish Women's Hospitals which included volunteers from Canada, Britain, Australia and several other nations.[9] The Scottish Women's Hospitals suffered enormously in Serbia and many of their doctors and nurses died before the campaign was over, including their founder and leader, Dr Elsie Inglis. She had organized the Scottish hospital group in Edinburgh in 1914, with the support of the Scottish suffrage societies who raised more than two million dollars to finance the project. Being patriots as well as fighters, the suffragettes had halted their personal battle to join the greater battle, but in spite of their patriotic enthusiasm and their successful fund-raising, the British Government initially refused the services of the Scottish Women's Hospitals. It seems incredible that such an offer should have been refused — fully equipped units, headed by fully qualified doctors — but this was early in the war, before things became too desperate, and the army didn't relish the idea of having to cope with groups of volunteer women, especially as many of them would be suffragettes.

Fortunately the allies weren't so particular, and the Scottish Women's Hospitals were soon established on the continent, doing invaluable work in Serbia, France, Belgium — wherever they were needed. So, too, was another group: the Women's Hospital Corps. This was also organized by suffragettes and its two leaders, Dr Flora Murray and Dr Louisa Garrett Anderson, were such renowned suffragettes that they didn't even bother to contact their own government. They offered their units directly to France and were given hospital space in the newly built Hotel Claridge in Paris. But it wasn't long before the British were asking for their services, suggesting that they establish a branch hospital at Wimereux; and in 1915 the Women's Hospital Corps was actually given charge of a military hospital at Endell Street in London. From then on, the work of all women doctors was gratefully accepted.

It would be hard to estimate how many women doctors served in the war, for they worked in such a variety of ways and for so many different nations that there is no comprehensive record. Three hundred and thirty-one are known to have been officially attached to the Royal Army Medical Corps (RAMC)[10] — of whom 85 served in Malta, 39 in Salonika, 36 in Egypt and 4 in France — but this doesn't by any means give a total count and neither, of course, does it indicate how many of them were Canadians. While some of our Canadian medical women were attached to the RAMC, others were actually commissioned in the Corps, with a rank and uniform. Many others worked separately from the War Office in various volunteer units. And some of them joined American units.

Dr Mary Lee Edward was one of those who joined an American unit.[11] She was an Ontario girl from Petrolea, a 1908 graduate from the University of Toronto, and the reason she joined an American rather than a Canadian or British group was that she was working

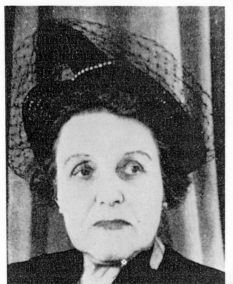

Dr Irma LeVasseur

Dr Mary Lee Edward in
lieutenant's uniform

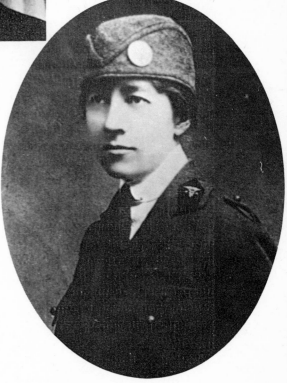

in New York when war broke out. She was one of our medical women who had left Canada because there wasn't the opportunity or scope for her here.

When she graduated in 1908, there was no Women's College Hospital, no real outlet for her talents, and she was both talented and ambitious. After graduating, she had been awarded a research scholarship at the University of Toronto — an exceptional honour — but it proved to be more of an honour than an opportunity. Dr Edward found herself in a backwater, a forgotten backwater. She hardly ever saw her supervisor, and when she realized that he was more interested in the latest play than in her research, she shook the snow from her boots and went off to the New York Infirmary for Women and Children. There she found all the opportunity she could hope for. First she was awarded a one thousand-dollar scholarship to study in Vienna, and then, after her return to New York, she was appointed House Physician (in other words, chief resident doctor) at the Infirmary.

When war broke out, Dr Edward had done several years' work at the Infirmary and she was to have experience in another New York hospital too. When America joined the war in 1917 and the men began to go overseas, she took over a man's job at New York's Hospital for Ruptured and Crippled, working in the operating theatre there. So she had surgical experience before she set to work on the battlefield.

It was towards the end of the war that she arrived on the battlefield, for it was only after America had entered the fighting that the women of the country began to organize on a large scale. Before then they hadn't felt the full impact, but by late 1917 the horror stories of life in the trenches were being heard so often and so personally that an increasing number of women began to feel that they must do something really active for the boys up there at the Front.

Two of the most concerned were Dr Edward and her American friend, Dr Caroline Finley, who was also from the Women's Infirmary. Between them, and with the backing of the Infirmary, they organized the Women's Overseas Hospitals, which were to be similar to the Scottish Women's Hospitals, and which were also supported by suffrage associations. Dr Finley and Dr Edward were in the first unit to go overseas and they went straight to France. It was all arranged with the French representatives in New York, so they knew exactly where they were going and in what capacity: they had been assigned to the 'devastated area' (the area that had already been fought over) and they were to run a hospital for women and children there, thus releasing the hospital's male staff for active service.

However, they never reached the devastated area. They had only got as far as Paris when they heard that their hospital had been bombed out of existence. But there they were in France, a fully equipped unit, far too valuable to be overlooked, so they were asked if they would go to the Front as part of the Tenth French Army.

This was not a welcome suggestion to all the ladies. Some of them suddenly remembered that they had pressing business at home — and one young lady, who couldn't bring herself to face the front line, offered the sturdier characters a small bunch of violets (as a substitute for her war service!). There had been about thirty women in the original unit: four doctors, several graduate nurses and quite a number of well-born but untrained young ladies who had volunteered as ambulance drivers or aides, or whatever was needed. About half of these returned home. But the strong stayed on, and among the strong were the four lady doctors: Dr Finley, who was head of the unit, Dr Edward, Dr Von Sholly and Dr Pavitsky.

Dr Pavitsky didn't remain at the Front. Her training was in pathology and there wasn't much use for a pathologist on a battle-field. But the other three doctors were well qualified for the work. Both Mary Lee Edward and Caroline Finley had already practised as surgeons, and Anna Von Sholly had experience as an anaesthetist.

They were sent to the Château Ognon at Senlis, right up at the Front, and they arrived there in time to receive the full brunt of the great German offensive of the spring and summer of 1918. This was no sinecure job. Often the hospital was attacked from the air by bombs or strafed by machine-gun fire. But the lady doctors were too busy to notice much of what was happening around them. Dr Edward was immediately assigned to the operating theatre to work with a French army surgeon, and Dr Finley not only operated but was also put in charge of her own barracks.

At times their patients would arrive by the hundred, wheeled down on stretchers into the preparation room where they would be cleaned of mud and grass by Miss Mackenzie, an American graduate nurse, and then on they would go to the American anaesthetist and to the Canadian, French or American surgeon. It was a thoroughly international team as well as being a co-sexual one. But the work was grim.

On more than one occasion, when the doctors went off duty, they would realize that they had been working alongside a whole box of legs that they had amputated during the night. There wasn't time for any attention to delicacies, no time to talk of shielding ladies from the grosser side of life. Sometimes Dr Edward operated for as long as sixty hours at a stretch, not pausing to sleep and hardly pausing to eat. Shells burst around her, bombs fell on the hospital ('thirteen nurses killed, eleven wounded'), and on she went, cutting and stitching.

'Operated 12 midnight to 8 A.M.' reads her diary. 'Operated 4-12 P.M. There remained 100 wounded to operate on. At times there are 400 or more arriving all the time. . . . Boche advancing. . . . Operating now with three equipes. . . . Evacuating and operating at high speed. Some on tables four hours after wounded. . . . Many evacuants from Compeigne. . . .'[12]

She was exhausted, and yet there was no stopping. She couldn't stop as long as the casualties kept coming in. And the casualties poured in until later in the year when at last the war turned in favour of the allies.

Before the war ended, the three lady doctors (as well as the graduate nurse, Miss Mackenzie) were all awarded the Croix de Guerre. It was bestowed on them at a special ceremony held at the Front, and one feels that the medals were given then, rather than later, because there was every chance that the French Government would only have been able to express its gratitude posthumously if it had waited any longer. But Dr Edward did survive the war — and much more too. She had already survived typhoid, which she had contracted when performing typhoid tests at the Women's Infirmary in New York, and she was later to survive being struck by lightning on a mountaineering holiday in Colorado. She was a true, tough Canadian, and with the sturdy spirit of her kind she went on practising medicine until she was eighty-five years old.

After the war, the University of Toronto awarded Dr Edward a Roll of Service in honour of her gallant work 'for our King and Country'. This was only fitting, but it strikes rather an odd note when one considers that she was serving in a unit enlisted in republican America and that she was working for republican France in a French military hospital and as part of the French army. Another anomaly was that while Dr Edward had great difficulty in speaking French, she was very fluent in German, the language of the enemy. This was because of her year in Vienna, and she continued to like the Austrians while hating the Germans. The whole contrariness of her position makes her characteristic of the women who served in the war: a Canadian in the Tenth French Army, paid by an organization in America, hating the Boche (in whose language she was fluent), loving the Austrians and serving with the French, while wearing a uniform which had been designed in the United States.

The uniform was a khaki skirt and jacket with red tabs, but here too there were contradictions. Although Dr Edward was formally termed 'lieutenant', as a woman she held no official rank and she was generally called 'miss' or 'mademoiselle'. It was a thorough mix-up.

A young woman who gave rise to almost as many irregularities was Dr Frances Evelyn Windsor, who was gazetted into the Canadian army. According to the *Canadian Medical Association Journal*,[13] she was the first woman physician ever to receive an appointment with the Canadian Army Medical Corps. She joined up in 1916 and one of the reasons that she managed to do so was that R.B. Bennett, at that time a member of the federal parliament, was deeply in love with her. Evelyn Windsor might have managed it anyway — she was a true-blue patriot, a staunch royalist and she *knew* that she must serve overseas — but undoubtedly R.B. Bennett's support helped her to do so.

However, his influence doesn't seem to have extended as far as the ship that was to take her overseas. Nobody on board was expecting a woman passenger: Frances Evelyn (not necessarily a woman's name), serving with the Canadian Army Medical Corps (obviously male). There was consternation when Miss Windsor mounted the gangway. Somebody would have to vacate a cabin!

This type of mistake happened so often that, within a few months, she was transferred to the British Army. Of course, the position of women with the British forces was also irregular, but at least Dr Windsor wasn't the only woman, and she was duly commissioned Captain, wearing a uniform whose jacket was identical with that of male officers.[14]

This proved to be fortunate on two counts, both of which were connected with her marriage — for Evelyn married in 1917. She married Edward Leacock (the brother of Stephen Leacock) who had also signed on with the British forces and had also been commissioned Captain. So she didn't outrank him. And, moreover, the couple could get by on three jackets instead of four — one each to wear, and one at the cleaners.

Evelyn did all her war service in England, working as an anaesthetist in the hospitals there, but in spite of her patriotism, it wasn't a very long service. As a newlywed, young Mrs Dr Captain Leacock very soon conceived a child — and this proved to be even more irregular than her commission in the army. When she applied for release because of her pregnancy, she discovered that the army *couldn't* release her. There was nothing in Army Regulations which allowed for such a contingency. As the months passed and as the day of her confinement approached, Evelyn began to get a little worried. She wasn't the type of woman to worry over trifles, but it did look as if her baby was going to be born while she was on duty. What was she going to *do?* What she did was to contract a mild case of pleurisy, though. not intentionally. But that was all right, pleurisy was an acceptable illness. Almost on the eve of her child's birth, Captain Windsor Leacock was released from the army on grounds of ill health — thus saving the RAMC the confusion of having a baby tangled in its red tape.

Eo Evelyn Windsor Leacock retired from the service, but of course she didn't retire from medicine. After she had returned to Canada and born a family of three children, she embarked on a second medical career which was no less unusual than her military service. For twenty years she served as the resident doctor and medical superintendent on the Blackfoot Indian Reserve at Gleichen outside Calgary. Certainly, other women doctors had worked among the Indians, but none had done so in the same capacity as Evelyn Windsor. She wasn't serving as a missionary or as the wife of a missionary or administrator. Her position was Medical Superintendent, and it was a position which previously had always been held by a man.

The significance of this appointment was not that Evelyn Windsor was a woman taking on a man's job, but that it was no longer considered extraordinary for a woman to do so. The war had brought changes in attitude, a new appraisal of the role of women in medicine. Sex was no longer the almost insurmountable barrier that it had been only a decade earlier.

SOME EARLY STAFF MEMBERS OF
THE WOMEN'S COLLEGE HOSPITAL

DOROTHEA JOHNSTON ORR (Trinity, 1899)

Dorothea Johnston Orr studied and graduated in medicine after her husband's death. She then interned in New York and worked there for some years. On returning to Toronto, Dr Orr established a practice for women and children, and she joined the staff of the Women's College Hospital. She died in 1946.

CAROLINE SOPHIA BROWN (Trinity, 1900)

Dr Brown taught school for many years before taking up medicine. After graduating from Trinity, she went on to do postgraduate work in Ireland and England and then returned to Toronto, where she ran a general practice for 25 years and where she joined the staff of the Women's College Hospital. She was a member of the Council of Women, of the IODE, of the Home and School Council and a member of the Ward Five Liberal-Conservative Association. She died in 1936.

MINERVA REID and HANNA REID (Toronto, 1905)

Both these sisters became doctors and both were connected with the Women's College Hospital. Minerva was one of the first members of its Board of Directors and was the hospital's Chief Surgeon between 1915 and 1925, while Hanna specialized as an anaesthetist and as an obstetrician. Often the sisters worked together at the hospital, Hanna administering the anaesthetic and Minerva performing the operation.

They came from a pioneering family of 12 children and were born and brought up near Orangeville, Ontario. Hanna died in 1955 and Minerva died in 1957.

ELIZABETH STEWART (Toronto, 1911)

Elizabeth Stewart was born near Uxbridge, Ontario, in 1890, and after graduating she interned at the Woman's Hospital in Philadelphia and then went on to do postgraduate work in radiology in New York. She was appointed radiologist at the Women's College Hospital, where she worked until 1956. She died in 1969.

HELEN BELL MILBURN (Toronto, 1919)
Helen Bell (Mrs Milburn) worked in the Radiology Department of the
Toronto General Hospital and then joined Dr Stewart at the Women's
College Hospital. Dr Milburn was Chief of the Out-Patients Department at
the Women's College Hospital and Chairman of the Breast Cancer Research
Committee there.

ETHEL HAYES (Toronto, 1912)
For many years Dr Hayes held the position of Chief of Medicine at the
Women's College Hospital. She was born in London, Ontario, in 1885 and
died in Toronto in 1971.

VETERANS OF THE FIRST WAR

MARGARET PARKS (Trinity, 1901)

Dr Parks came from Saint John, N.B., and practised there until she enlisted as a Nursing Sister with the RAMC in the First War. She served in France as a nursing sister and as an anaesthetist and, after the war, she worked as medical inspector for the Immigration Service of the Canadian Government. Later she took up public health work in Manitoba. She died in 1955.

E. VICTORIA REID SILVERTHORN (Queen's, 1904)

Victoria Reid (Mrs Silverthorn) graduated in Arts from Queen's in 1900 and then studied at the Ontario Medical College for Women, taking the medical exams of Queen's University. Queen's was still willing to grant women degrees, even though it was not accepting them as medical students. ADELAIDE TURNER (Queen's, 1897) also received a Queen's degree after pursuing her studies at the Ontario Medical College for Women. Dr Silverthorn interned in Boston after graduating in medicine, and she later joined the staff of the Women's College Hospital. She served for many years as a counsellor at Queen's University. During the First War, she was appointed to the staff of the London General Hospital in England. She died in 1949.

PEARL JANE SPROULE MANSON (Toronto, 1907)

Jane Sproule (Mrs Manson) took postgraduate studies in Toronto, Vienna and Berlin and was admitted to the Royal College of Physicians in London in 1911. She did her war service in London and on her return to Canada, she headed the otolaryngology department of the Women's College Hospital. She died in 1961.

LILY BOYINGTON MATHIESON (Toronto, 1909)

Lily Boyington (Mrs Mathieson) served with the Canadian Army Medical Corps in the First War. She was born in Kent County and she died in Kingston in 1966, at the age of 76. She was appointed to the staff of the Hospital for Sick Children, Toronto, and later she practised in Port Rowan. Dr Mathieson moved to Belleville when she was in her forties.

EDNA GUEST (Toronto, 1910)

Edna Guest covered many different fields and proved herself outstanding in all of them. After graduating from Toronto, she did postgraduate work at Harvard and interned at the Women's and Children's Hospital in Boston.

From 1912 to 1915, Dr Guest held the post of Professor of Anatomy and Assistant in Surgery as a missionary at the women's medical college in Ludhiana in India. On her way home from India during the First War, she joined the Scottish Women's Hospitals and was put in charge of the base hospital in Corsica. Returning to Canada after the war, she established a private practice in Toronto and she also became Chief of Surgery at the Women's College Hospital. In 1932 Dr Guest was awarded the OBE and in 1940-41, she held the position of President of the Federation of Medical Women of Canada.

ISOBEL DAY (Toronto, 1926)
Dr Day did her First War service as a nurse, before she had graduated in medicine. She served in France and England and was decorated for her gallantry with the Royal Red Cross. Dr Day also served in the Second World War — as a commissioner in the St John Ambulance Brigade. Dr Day had been a silver medalist in medicine from the University of Toronto and for many years was on the staff of the Vancouver General Hospital. In 1931-32 she was President of the Federation of Medical Women of Canada. She died in Vancouver in 1953.

10

Winning fame in the West

As a matter of fact, it is doubtful if Evelyn Windsor's sex had ever proved much of a barrier to her, even before the war. When she had first come to Calgary in 1911, the newspapers had heralded her arrival with the headline: 'Fair Fems Have All the Frills!' No opposition there. And there was no opposition from the medical men either. Evelyn had registered herself without difficulty at the College of Physicians and Surgeons and, without difficulty, she had established a small practice for women and children which she ran with Rosamond Leacock, her friend, classmate and future sister-in-law.[1]

The two young women were both University of Toronto graduates and they had decided to open a practice in Calgary because of the glowing reports of the city that they had received from one of the men in their year. There was opportunity there, a growing community, plenty of scope. In 1911, Calgary had a population of forty-four thousand and it was growing at the rate of a thousand a month. It was a boom town, charging energetically into the future and there was work for all who came, especially for women doctors, for although the Yeomans ladies had retired to Calgary a few years previously, there were no women practising medicine in the city. The novelty of having *two* pretty young ladies as doctors was therefore a very welcome event. Besides, they did have all the frills. After graduating from the University of Toronto in 1908, they had spent almost three years doing postgraduate work, interning and getting practical experience. They had been to Johns Hopkins in Baltimore, to the Woman's Medical College of Pennsylvania, the Hospital for Women in Detroit, and had then spent three months visiting hospitals in Europe.[2] They were very highly qualified, and Calgary was glad to receive them.

The only person who seems to have had any misgivings about their presence in the city was Rosamond's mother. She, too, had heard reports of Calgary, of Calgary the 'wide open' town with its Houses of Ill Fame and its hundreds of saloons and thousands of lusty young men. It was no place for young ladies of good family, especially such young and inexperienced ladies as Rosamond and Evelyn. Although they both had plenty of experience in the world of medicine, Mrs Leacock was keenly aware that they had very little experience of the world in general. They couldn't possibly live in Calgary unchaperoned. If they insisted on going there, then she would accompany them.

So the threesome — the two doctors and their chaperone — set up house in Calgary, which proved to be all that Mrs. Leacock had expected. Before long, the young doctors found it wise to inform the police whenever they were called to one of the more dubious parts of town. Maybe they were doctors, but they were also attractive young women, and a skirt was a skirt — as they discovered very quickly. But their practice went well and it had become encouragingly busy by the time Evelyn went off to the war in 1916.

Rosamond continued on her own while Evelyn was away, getting appointed to the School Board,[3] steadily increasing both her reputation and the number of her patients, and becoming well known as 'our Dr Leacock'. (Evelyn was always known as Dr Windsor, even after her marriage.) But Rosamond's chief interest was pathology and, in 1918, when the changing attitudes were already opening new opportunities for women, she decided to give up her practice and specialize in pathology. She set up the Calgary Clinical Laboratory, and at the same time she got herself appointed pathologist at two hospitals — the Calgary General and the Holy Cross.

All this was very promising for Rosamond, but it wasn't so promising for Evelyn when, in 1927, she came west again. By this time Evelyn had separated from her husband and although he was looking after the two older children, she had the care of the youngest, who was still a toddler. So she couldn't go into general practice on her own (how could she leave such a small child unattended if she was called out on an emergency?); a year's hospital work in Montreal hadn't proved satisfactory either, in spite of its more regular hours. She could have done with a shared practice with a good friend like Rosamond. But Rosamond was specializing in pathology now. Evelyn was on her own.

She wasn't on her own for very long. She had plenty of friends in Calgary who had been impressed by her work when she was the young Fair Fem doctor. First she was offered a job with the Calgary Public School Board and this was soon followed by the offer of work at Gleichen, on the Blackfoot Reserve, first in a temporary capacity and then, in 1928, as the Medical Superintendent. It was the perfect post for Evelyn. She was given a house on the reserve (so that solved accommodation problems) and, since she was provided with a nursing staff, someone would always be around to keep an eye on her child when she was called out. Rations were also provided — the same rations as were provided to the Blackfoot — and these were to stand her in good stead during the depression. When she first took the job, few doctors were interested in it — the salary was small and, besides, it didn't *lead* anywhere — but during the thin years, her position was eyed enviously. What right had a woman to be sitting so pretty when there were men in need? On more than one occasion, attempts were made to remove her from the reserve, but they all failed: Dr Windsor was a war veteran, so she couldn't be turned out of her job.

Although the Gleichen appointment was not the most coveted of jobs when she was first offered it, that wasn't the reason why she was offered it. She was sought out for the job because the reserve badly needed a woman doctor (the Indians wouldn't let their wives be examined by male doctors). And she, particularly, was felt to be the right woman doctor because she had already gained a reputation in Calgary, both before the war and since her return, as a pragmatic and capable woman who was unshockably down-to-earth. She had been an outspoken supporter of Calgary's 'red light' district — so much more hygienic to keep it all in one place — and it was felt that if she could speak out so boldly at committee meetings while the men were humming and hawing and trying to discuss prostitution without mentioning any words that *meant* anything (because there was a lady present), then she would also be able to cope with the

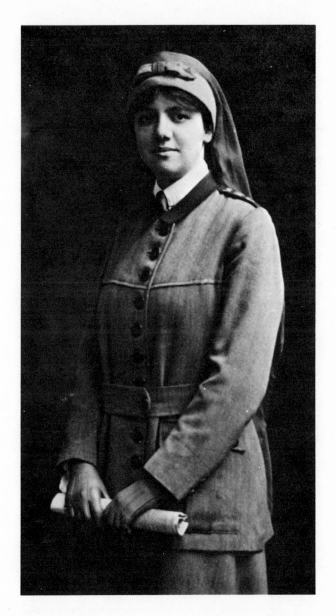

Dr Evelyn Windsor when she joined the army

challenging problems that she would encounter on an Indian reserve. And she wouldn't be frightened of living alone there. Dr
Windsor might look elegantly genteel, but there was a solid core
beneath her beauty.

There was also an open-mindedness, a willingness to accept that
different people had different values. Her relationship with the
Blackfoot was based on mutual respect. She respected their ancient
lore and their customs and, in their turn, they respected her for her
respect of them. She wouldn't have been able to achieve nearly so
much with her medical work if she hadn't established this healthy
relationship with her patients. She made a point of learning their
tribal traditions and, when her older children came to visit, she
made sure that they too observed the conventions and treated
Blackfoot customs with dignity.

This was important as well as thoughtful, for when Dr Windsor
first went to Gleichen, the Indian people there were still living very
much in their old ways, believing in their own gods, worshipping
the sun, holding their annual Tobacco Dance in the spring and
their Sun Dance at midsummer. Although missionaries had been
at work on the reserve for a good many decades, and although they
had succeeded in opening schools and in getting the women to dress
with becoming modesty, they had had very little success spiritually.
As late as 1933 they were writing, rather sorrowfully, that the religion of the Blackfoot, 'like all ancient faiths, is very resistant to
Christianity.'[4]

However, this was not the concern of Evelyn Windsor. She was
not a missionary. Although she was a practising Anglican and the
daughter of an Anglican clergyman, she didn't see why the Blackfoot should also be turned into Anglicans. They had their own
religion and it worked very well for them — in fact, it worked un-
cannily well at times. People who shouldn't have recovered from an
illness did sometimes recover, just because of their faith in their
own medicine men. It happened too often to be discounted. And
those who were ready to die, did die.

On one occasion, a very old member of the tribe came to say
goodbye to Dr Windsor because he was going to die at three o'clock
that afternoon. Evelyn wasn't as sceptical as her medical degree
might have made her. Although the man was in good health, she
wished him *bon voyage* on his long journey, and stood with his

friends and relatives while he smoked his last pipe and then wrapped himself in a blanket and settled comfortably into his coffin. He died peacefully and expectedly on the exact stroke of three. Unsurprised, Dr Windsor observed the formalities with his surviving relatives, and then returned to the hospital to treat the living who had not yet decided to die.

A small hospital had been established on the reserve in 1922, but it had never received any women patients before Evelyn Windsor took charge of it.[5] Nor had it been very popular with the men. It wasn't so much that the sparkling hygiene of the hospital had alarmed them — their own teepees were always kept very clean — it was more the unfamiliarity of the surroundings that kept them away and the fact that the patients were made to sleep in beds. They weren't used to beds: they were frightened they would fall out in the night. And the women were frightened on another count: although the nurses were female, the doctors had always been male. Babies had therefore been born at home, in teepee or hut, and many of them had also died at home. The infant mortality rate had been pathetically high.

Not so once Dr Windsor took charge. From then on, all babies were born in the hospital, and before each mother left the hospital, she was given a complete layette of clothing, plus instruction. Baby clinics were started, educational baby shows were given, the children became healthier and chubbier, and many more of them survived those dangerous first years. All except twins. Twins were considered unlucky, and however much Dr Windsor nurtured or fostered them, one of them always died. In an attempt to break this tradition (a custom she couldn't approve of), she kept one pair of twins for what seemed a safe period. One of the twins was returned home after a year, without any ill effect, and the other wasn't returned home until it was three years old. Even so, it died almost immediately.

Although much of Dr Windsor's work at Gleichen was concerned with women and children, as Medical Superintendent she was in charge of the health of all the Blackfoot on the reserve and she spent a large portion of her early years there trying to reduce the incidence of tuberculosis. Like so many other Indian tribes, the Blackfoot were being ravaged by tuberculosis, the 'white man's disease' that was reducing their numbers even more drastically than the destruction of the buffalo had done. Sometimes a whole family would all have TB, the children dying one by one, the younger being infected by their older brothers and sisters. Although there was no cure for TB when Dr Windsor started work at Gleichen, there was at least prevention, and she started an energetic campaign with regular X-rays, moving the sick out of their family groups and into sanitoriums and successfully controlling the spread of the disease.

A less routine type of work that she also had to cope with was the occasional mining accident. There was a small coal mine on the re-serve, and every so often a man would be trapped or crushed and the doctor would be called. Dr Windsor hated going down the mine, especially when part of it had just fallen in and another fall was more than a possibility. But down she would go, concealing her fear. It simply wouldn't do to let the Indians see that she was afraid.

In spite of Evelyn Windsor's observance of Blackfoot customs, there was a touch of the Raj in her. She took it for granted that she belonged to a superior race and she knew that she must maintain her superiority in all circumstances. Straight backed, dignified, and very much the lady, she was the authority, the doctor, the one who gave orders and issued instructions and *told* the Blackfoot how they ought to behave. She drew their admiration, their gratefulness and their affection — but she didn't invite familiarity.

Nor did she shrug her shoulders philosophically when her orders were disobeyed. On one occasion she was furious to find that one of her patients — a woman who had given birth to a child only a few hours earlier — was energetically putting up a teepee at the Calgary Stampede. It was bad, stupid and disobedient and Dr Windsor told the mother so. She should have been resting up for ten days as she had been instructed to do. She shouldn't even be in Calgary. The city was about fifty miles away from Gleichen and, to get there by buckboard, the mother must have set off almost as soon as her baby had been born.

The Indian mother might have known that her presence in Cal-gary would have been discovered: Dr Windsor always visited the Blackfoot encampment when she was at the stampede. After all, the Blackfoot were friends as well as patients and although the friendship was based on respect, it was a very real friendship. Even after Dr Windsor retired, she only had to appear at the stampede to be surrounded by members of the band, who would proudly show her their growing children, enquire after her family and hospitably invite her into their teepees to talk over old times. Leaving a teepee one afternoon, when she had taken her small granddaughter to the stampede, Dr Windsor found herself being stared at curiously by a couple of American tourists.

'My! They do dress them well!' said the wife.

Dr Windsor smiled. She must have got more sunburned than she had realized. But the remark wasn't so inappropriate: by this time she had been made an honorary member of the Blackfoot tribe. She was to receive other honours too. Although Dr Windsor's work took place far away from the main thrust of world events in a remote stretch of flat prairie fifty miles beyond Calgary, it didn't pass unnoticed. In 1937, she was awarded the Coronation Medal of King George VI.

In the meantime her sister-in-law, Rosamond Leacock, had also been gaining an impressive reputation. She had left Calgary and returned to Toronto, where she was well known in musical circles as well as medical circles, for she had graduated from the Toronto Conservatory of Music as well as graduating in medicine, and she retained her interest in music. But, of course, pathology was her main subject. For many years she worked as assistant to Dr I.H. Erb in the bacteriology department of Toronto's Hospital for Sick Children, and when Dr Erb was made Provincial Pathologist, Rosamond moved on with him, becoming Assistant to the Provincial Pathologist.

Pathology was a relatively new opening for women, in spite of Maude Abbott's specialization in the subject, but in the years after the war quite a number of medical women had entered this branch of medicine and several of them had been given government appointments. Dr Lola McLatchie had been appointed Provincial Pathologist for Alberta, and next door, in Saskatchewan, a woman was also taken on as Provincial Pathologist. This was Dr Frances McGill, whose work as Provincial Pathologist proved so valuable that she was given a most singular appointment: she was made a member of the Royal Canadian Mounted Police.

Most of Dr McGill's obituaries record with pride that she was the only woman who ever served with the Royal Canadian Mounted Police, but in fact the RCMP did hire women from time to time, in

minor capacities as non-uniformed assistants.[6] However, Dr Mc-
Gill's role was anything but minor. As Honorary Surgeon at the
RCMP Laboratory in Regina, and as lecturer in forensic medicine at
the police college classes, she was a key figure in the Force, a well
known and very popular member of the Regina Depot.

She was appointed Honorary Surgeon with the Mounties in
1946,[7] right at the end of her career and after her retirement from
the post of Provincial Pathologist, but her association with the Force
had begun long before then. For nearly twenty years, Dr McGill
had been working closely with the police, analysing specimens, performing autopsies, dissecting and detecting — and solving almost
as many mysteries as Maigret. Her honorary appointment was a
token of gratitude for past services as much as a contract for future
service. It was an acknowledgement of what she already was: one
of the Mounties.

'All she really lacked was the uniform,' said one of her associates.
This was true. After all, Dr McGill was on the RCMP payroll — she
received a token salary — and she was also appropriately Mounty
in her habits: she was a keen horsewoman. She kept two horses, one
of whom (she said) would stop dead in its tracks at the mention of
Mackenzie King. Dr McGill was a staunch Conservative.[8]

She was staunch in every way, a short and rather solid woman,
solid mentally as well as physically, meticulous in her work and
entirely dependable. For she wasn't out to save or blame: she only
wanted to discover the truth. Naturally the police greatly appreciated these qualities, just as they appreciated her briskness, her
matter-of-fact attitude to the most gory crimes. But most of all they
appreciated the thoroughness of her investigations. If Dr McGill
said that the evidence was conclusive, then you could be sure that
it was. It would hold up in court.

Frances McGill used to give an impressive performance in court.
A small, upright figure, who couldn't be inveigled into saying something she didn't mean, she used to stand to give her evidence (the
men weren't offered a chair, so why should she sit?) always wearing
a hat as a sign of respect, and speaking with a preciseness which
delighted the police. Only occasionally was an opposing Counsel
foolish enough to ask her leading questions — and then he generally wished he hadn't. Once, when she was asked a series of questions which were growing increasingly insulting — for instance,

'had she removed the clothing before performing the autopsy?' (of course she had! she would hardly dissect a cadaver with its clothes on!) — she was finally asked if she had searched the victim's pockets.

'That is the role of the legal profession,' replied Dr McGill icily. But normally her evidence was given with the utmost politeness, for she had a great sense of decorum. Her associates on the Force admired her, as much as anything, for being 'a real lady'.

This seems rather a strange epithet when one considers that Frances McGill wasn't the most feminine type of woman. She was gruff and rather hearty, a great favourite around the Regina Depot because she would answer quip for quip, just like a male colleague. Yet although the men enjoyed her quick wit and her good-humoured camaraderie, they were very conscious that she was a *lady* officer. They might treat her almost as a male colleague, making no allowances for fatigue — and being expected to make none — when they were driving hundreds of miles on a case, but they were very proud of 'Doc' and very fond of her, and when they were off duty, or not in the thick of a case, they took pleasure in showing their admiration with kindly gallantries. Very often there were pleasantries too. For instance, when the doctor asked a group of them to her apartment for a cocktail, the jokes flew. It was inevitable.

'Ice?' she would ask.

'Please.'

She would open the door of her refrigerator, and there, side by side with the milk would be a selection of sealed bottles. This one might have a human heart in it, the next one a kidney. . . . The refrigerator was the storeroom for whatever Dr McGill happened to be working on that week.

Of course most of her work was done in the laboratory, either the provincial laboratory or the RCMP laboratory, but if she was absorbingly interested in a specimen, she might take it home to work on in the evening. Part of the reason why she was so successful in criminal work was that the detective aspects intrigued her as much as the medical, and once she had started to puzzle out a mystery, she just had to inspect and think and inspect again until she came up with the answer. The only possible answer.

Dr McGill had been interested in law, and had even studied it, before she had decided to specialize in medicine. She was thirty-

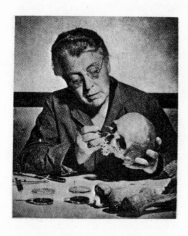

Dr Frances McGill at work (left) and mounted (below, on left)

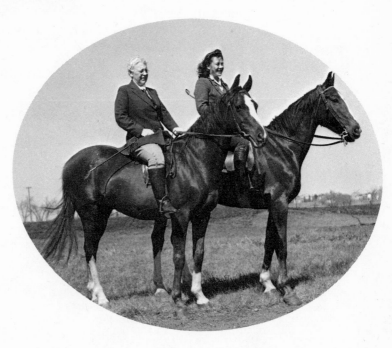

seven before she graduated as a doctor, though this wasn't entirely because of her law studies. Education was an expensive business and her family wasn't rich. She was a Manitoba girl, brought up on a farm in Minnedosa, and like many other women doctors before her, she had been obliged to teach school for several years in order to put herself through college. College was the Manitoba Medical College from which she graduated in 1915, winning the gold medal for the highest scholastic average, the Dean's prize for general proficiency and a prize in surgical history. After a year's internship at the Winnipeg General Hospital and a couple of years at the Manitoba Provincial Laboratory, Dr McGill took the post of Provincial Bacteriologist in the Saskatchewan Department of Health. This was her stepping-stone and a few years later she was appointed Provincial Pathologist for Saskatchewan and Laboratory Director.

In 1922, when Dr McGill first took on the post of Provincial Pathologist, the RCMP laboratory hadn't yet been established, so all the forensic medicine was done in the provincial laboratory. And it was done by Frances McGill. At first it was done for the provincial police, later for the RCMP, but later still *by* the RCMP. In 1938 the Mounties established their own laboratory at the Regina Depot[9] and Dr McGill found, to her disappointment, that her services were no longer required. Curious and criminal cases were all referred to Dr Maurice Powers, an RCMP Surgeon who had been appointed especially to set up and run the Depot's laboratory. This was in no way a slur on Dr McGill's work. It was simply that the Force was growing and that it needed its own forensic laboratory with its own staff. Relations remained amicable, and in 1943 when Dr Powers was killed in a plane crash, she was called in to take over his work.

By this time Dr McGill was sixty-six. She had retired from her post as Provincial Pathologist the previous year and had opened a practice in Regina specializing in allergies and skin diseases. But of course she was only too glad to help her old friends, the Mounties, and even though she continued her practice and only worked part-time for the RCMP, it was always wholeheartedly.

Just how many criminals were convicted because of Dr McGill's work would be hard to assess, but she seems to have released the innocent as often as nailing the guilty. In one case — the Lintlaw Case — the police were sure that they had their man. There couldn't be any doubt. A young man had been found dead in his shack, shot through the head, and the murder weapon (a rifle) had been found carefully hidden in a bin of wheat beside his bed. There was blood everywhere in the shack, on the walls, on the floor, all over the victim's face (obviously there had been a real bust-up before the shooting) and there were also plenty of bloodstains on the fur coat of a neighbouring farmer. It was as simple as two and two make four. The neighbouring farmer was arrested. Naturally he *said* that the blood on his coat was animal blood, that one of his calves had cut its ear and he had wrapped it in his coat to keep it warm. But that type of story had been heard before. Obviously it was a straightforward murder case. The police discovered that the victim had borrowed the rifle from a friend in order to go crow-shooting — but instead of shooting crows he must have got into a fight with his neighbour and ended up by being shot himself. No mystery here. All the same, Dr McGill was called in: it was routine procedure to consult her in homicide cases.

It was also routine procedure for Dr McGill to question the evidence, however watertight it seemed. Why were the police so sure that this was murder? The local doctor had said that death was instantaneous, but how did he know? How carefully had he examined the body? There was nothing in his report which explained the immediacy of the man's death. In fact the report wasn't nearly detailed enough for Frances McGill's fastidious accuracy, so she decided to have the body exhumed and to examine it herself.

The first thing she discovered was that the 'victim' couldn't possibly have been murdered. Only he could have fired a rifle so that the bullet pierced his head at that particular angle: the bullet had entered under his chin and gone straight up. This being the case, he would have lived for some time after shooting himself, so if he didn't want his death to look like suicide, he would have had time to hide the rifle before he died, and he would also have been able to daub himself with blood, as if he had been fighting. And since he could have moved around his shack, there was no mystery about how it had become so bloodstained.

Once Dr McGill began reasoning on these lines, there was plenty more to be rechecked. The neighbour who had lent the rifle — his story should be heard again. It was very interesting. Apparently the young 'victim' had initially asked for only one bullet when he

borrowed the rifle. Only one? To go crow-shooting? Meantime
the accused's coat was being analysed. Animal blood, he had said.
And it was animal blood. And his calf did have a cut on its ear. The
suspect was released. Dr McGill had done it again.

Of course, many of Frances McGill's investigations did support
the police theories — she wasn't always pulling a rabbit out of a
hat — but on a great many occasions it was her theories alone, followed by her careful and very logical analyses, which eventually
led to release or conviction. The story of these cases makes fascinat-
ing reading.[10] There was the Bran Muffin Case in which a woman
tried to poison her father and succeeded in killing her grandparents
instead — a crime apparently without motive and not suspected as
a crime until Dr McGill got busy on it. There was the Elzie Burden
Case in which a local boy — and not a migrant worker — was found
to be the murderer. There was the South Poplar Case which wasn't
murder at all. The apparent victim had died of a heart attack. It
was the angle at which the body lay, plus the below-freezing
weather, plus the fact that he suffered from ricketts which had
caused his head to look as if it had been bashed in. Over the years
hundreds and probably thousands of cases were solved by Frances
McGill — by her genius for detection as much as by her careful
medical investigations.

She was certainly a most remarkable woman and when she died,
at the age of eighty-one, it wasn't only the RCMP who remembered
her with gratitude. She had made a name for herself throughout
the West, and it was only natural that the Province of Saskatchewan
should decide to honour her memory. It did so by naming a lake
after her. On April 3, 1959, a few months after Frances McGill's
death, McGill Lake, north of Lake Athabasca, was officially marked
on the map.[11]

The significance of this action was appropriately symbolic, a sign
not only of Frances McGill's status but of the status of all our
women. For there was no longer any doubt about the position of
medical women in Canada. No longer were they considered of value
only in certain areas. Literally as well as figuratively women doctors
were firmly on the map.

SOME POST-WAR GRADUATES

ELLA PEARL HOPGOOD (Dalhousie, 1920)

Dr Hopgood came from Prince Edward Island. She specialized in psychiatry and was well known for her work with the mentally ill. In 1928 she was appointed Assistant Superintendent of the Nova Scotia Hospital and, due to her work with the St John Ambulance Association, she was made a Commander of the Order of St John. Dr Hopgood was one of the early members of the Federation of Medical Women of Canada and she served as president in 1928-29. She died in Dartmouth in 1957.

MABEL PATTERSON (Dalhousie, 1921)

Dr Patterson was also a President of the Federation of Medical Women of Canada (1938-39). She was a general practitioner and obstetrician in the Maritimes.

GLADYS STORY CUNNINGHAM (Manitoba, 1923)

Gladys Story (Mrs Cunningham) was born in Manitoba and she trained as a nurse before taking up medicine. She became engaged to a medical missionary while she was studying medicine and in 1923 (after winning the University of Manitoba's Gold Medal in Surgery) she went to China where she stayed, apart from home leave, until 1951. She and her husband then practised in Vancouver until their retirement in 1962. In China, Dr Cunningham worked mostly in Chengtu, teaching at the West China Union University and working in the Methodist hospitals. She died in Vancouver in 1972.

LOLA McLATCHIE (Toronto, 1922)

Dr McLatchie took over from Rosamond Leacock in Calgary, specializing in pathology. She was Pathologist at the Calgary General Hospital, at the Red Cross Hospital for Children and was appointed Legal Pathologist for the Province of Alberta.

ADA WILSON WALLACE (Manitoba, 1922)

Ada Wilson (Mrs Wallace) interned at the Misericordia Hospital in Winnipeg before graduating. She married a minister and went with him to Herb Lake — being called out three times on her honeymoon. In 1939 the Wallaces moved to Emerson, Manitoba. Here Dr Wallace was the only doctor in the neighbourhood, and she acted as coroner as well as general practitioner. In 1950 she and her husband moved to Vancouver.

LILLIAN CHASE (Toronto, 1922)

Dr Chase was a Nova Scotian by birth, but she worked in Regina for many years, specializing in diabetes and being appointed President of the medical staff of the Regina General Hospital. In the Second World War she served with the RCAMC and, after the war, while maintaining her connection with the militia, she held hospital appointments in Toronto.

SARA MELTZER (Manitoba, 1924)

Dr Meltzer became Assistant Pathologist to the Winnipeg General Hospital and Lecturer in Pathology at the University of Manitoba. She gained a reputation for her skill in tissue diagnosis and when she died in 1942, the University of Manitoba established a scholarship in her memory.

LATER GRADUATES

DOROTHEA MELLOR FRICKER (McGill, 1930)

Dr Mellor (Mrs Fricker) was associated with the Royal Victoria Hospital, Montreal, where she was physician to the nurses. In 1943-44 she was President of the Federation of Medical Women of Canada.

ROBERTA BOND NICHOLS (Dalhousie, 1925)

Roberta Bond (Mrs Nichols) first practised in Newfoundland, but she returned to Halifax when she married. After her husband's death, she joined the staff of Dalhousie University, becoming Lecturer in Anatomy and Associate Professor of Anaesthesiology, and also working as an anaesthetist in the Halifax hospitals. Dr Bond Nichols was President of the Federation of Medical Women of Canada 1958-59 and, on her death in 1966, the Nova Scotia branch of the Federation honoured her with the Roberta Bond Nichols Memorial. Dalhousie has named the departmental library in Anatomy the 'Roberta Bond Nichols Collection' and it also awards an annual prize in her name, which is given to a woman medical student.

AGNES MOFFAT MAGEE (McGill, 1931)

Dr Moffat (Mrs Magee) was born in Weston, Ontario in 1905. She interned at the Toronto General Hospital and also at hospitals in Michigan and Guelph, and between 1934 and 1936 she did postgraduate work in London and Vienna. She specialized in anaesthesia and paediatrics and joined the Peterborough Clinic, where she worked from 1936 to 1973. Dr Moffat was President of the Federation of Medical Women of Canada 1948-49.

MARGARET STRANG SAVAGE (Western Ontario, 1929)

Margaret Strang (Mrs Savage) was well known in the West as a horse-riding, frontier, missionary doctor. Born in Huron County, Ontario, in 1901, her first missionary posting was to Dixonville in the Peace River District. After her marriage, she moved to Cold Lake, Alberta. In 1965 she was given an honorary LL D by the University of Western Ontario. She died in 1970.

CLARA CHRISTIE MIGHT (McGill, 1925) and PEARL CHRISTIE DOWLING (McGill, 1927)

These sisters both taught school before taking up medicine and it was Clara, the younger of the two, who first decided to become a physician. She externed at the Montreal General Hospital on the surgical staff and then did a year at the Yale University Hospital, New Haven, specializing in obstetrics and gynaecology. Clara Christie opened a general practice in Calgary in 1927, working there through the depression — when she sometimes earned as little as $27 a week. Many of her patients couldn't afford doctors' fees, and if they paid Dr Christie at all, it was by making her a table or giving her a few vegetables.

During the Second World War, Clara (Mrs Might) was joined by Pearl (Mrs Dowling) who had been working in Detroit. They ran a joint practice in Calgary, Clara doing the obstetrics and Pearl the paediatrics. Pearl Christie Dowling held the office of President of the Federation of Medical Women of Canada, 1952-53.

ELINOR BLACK (Manitoba, 1930)
For thirteen years, Dr Black headed the Department of Obstetrics and Gynaecology at the University of Manitoba and in 1961 she was elected President of the Society of Obstetricians and Gynaecologists of Canada. In 1933 she was appointed to the staff of the Winnipeg General Hospital and she was also consultant to the St Boniface, Grace and Children's hospitals. She was born in Nelson, B.C. and went to school in Calgary before becoming a medical student at the University of Manitoba.

11

On the map

FIGURATIVELY, women doctors had been getting on the map ever
since the First World War. Their 'gallant service in winning the
war' had been the pretext on which McGill University finally
admitted them as medical students, and it was their indispensable
war service in so many fields which induced most of the professions
to lower the barriers and acknowledge that women could function
very well in men's jobs. It therefore seems strange that it was after
the war, when women were already beginning to share male privileges, that the Federation of Medical Women of Canada was
formed.

But the Federation was not a feminist organization, not pri-
marily. It wasn't intended to be an agitation group that would fight
with all its strength for women's rights. It was intended more as a
society through which women physicians from different provinces
— and different countries — could meet. Its original constitution
states that it was established 'to promote the welfare and interest
of medical women of Canada and of the Medical Profession and to
co-operate with the British Medical Women's Federation and with
similar Federations in other countries having like objects and
policy.'[1]

Both Britain and the United States already had a medical women's federation and, in 1920, the Medical Women's International
Association had been formed.[2] It had been formed largely to continue friendships which had been begun during the war. But Cana-

dian women doctors had also served in the war and, until they created a national society, they had no means of joining the International Association. They had no body which could foster the interchange of ideas, no organization through which women, working in the same field, could meet and discuss their work. Although many of our women doctors were members of the Canadian Medical Association, this didn't really fill the same role, for the CMA was composed mostly of men. It didn't have the same interest in the women's problems. And of course it had neither the desire nor the qualifications for membership in the Medical Women's International Association.

Obviously, Canada's women physicians needed their own society and, in 1924, a group of them decided to organize it. They had gathered in Ottawa for the meeting of the Canadian Medical Association and, at the CMA garden party, they moved off to a quiet piece of lawn, settled themselves on the grass, and began to plan. The chief planner was Dr Maude Abbott, who had naturally come to Ottawa for the CMA meeting.

Dr Abbott acted as Chairman at the Federation's organizing meeting that was held a few days later. There were six women present at this meeting[3] and, between them, they were a representative cross-section of the type of women in the medical profession. There was Maude Abbott, an internationally known figure. There was Helen MacMurchy, also famous internationally and one of the few women working in a senior position with the Federal Government. Then there was Elizabeth Bagshaw. Dr Bagshaw had been in general practice since 1906, but she wasn't a run-of-the-mill general practitioner. Already she was advocating birth control and she was to become medical adviser to Canada's first birth-control clinic, which she helped to organize in Hamilton. Jennie Smillie, another committee member, was a surgeon. A 1909 graduate from the University of Toronto, she had, at first, had difficulty finding a place to practise as a surgeon — her first operation in Canada had been performed in a private home — but since the establishment of the Women's College Hospital, she had been able to work in more suitable surroundings.

One surgeon, one academic, one government welfare officer and one pioneer in birth control. Inevitably the other two would be in general practice, and in fact both were longtime general practitioners. Janet Hall was an 1899 graduate of Trinity, and Elizabeth Embury was an 1888 graduate from Queen's, one of the very first women to graduate in medicine in Canada. All that was really lacking were missionaries — and of course they were out in the field — but many missionaries did join as the Federation grew. It grew very quickly. By the following year there were sixty-five charter members, including vice-presidents from Prince Edward Island, Nova Scotia, New Brunswick, Quebec, Ontario, Manitoba, Saskatchewan, Alberta and British Columbia.[4] Only the Northwest Territories and Newfoundland weren't represented (and of course Newfoundland hadn't yet joined Confederation).

Over the years, the membership continued to grow in spite of or, perhaps, because of the fact that more and more women were joining the Canadian Medical Association. The Federation's meetings were always arranged to coincide with the CMA meetings so that women attending one meeting could also attend the other. This is significant, because it shows that, even when it was formed, the Federation wasn't intended as an alternative to the CMA. It was simply a different gathering specially for women.

Although the Federation was feminine, rather than feminist, it did grow to become a form of guardian to our medical women. It has acted as guardian in several ways: by giving scholarships and student loans to promising women students and also, when necessary, by acting as a power group in dealing with problems which were of no great concern to the CMA, but which were of crucial importance to women doctors. During the Second World War, when women were needed in the services even more than they had been in the First War, the Federation saw to it that women physicians entered the forces on an appropriate footing.

In spite of Captain Evelyn Windsor's service with the Canadian Army Medical Corps in the 1914-18 war, no woman could legally be commissioned in any of Canada's armed forces until 1942 when a special Act of Parliament was passed. But the Act wasn't all that satisfactory as far as women physicians were concerned. They discovered that they would be expected to serve only with the women's forces, examining only women, serving in a subsidiary role to male physicians (some of whom might have been their classmates); that they would probably be of lower rank and that they would certainly get a lower salary.

'Out of the question,' said the Federation.

So a meeting was arranged with Brigadier Gorsseline, a representative of the army, in order to get more reasonable terms. It was quite an amicable meeting, but it sounds as if the brigadier didn't stand much of a chance against the Federation's committee. According to the Minutes of the meeting, there was 'a good deal of discussion . . . re. rank, duties, accommodation, dress, etc.' and then Brigadier Gorsseline agreed that women physicians would be commissioned in the Royal Canadian Army Medical Corps on the same terms as male physicians, with equal rank and pay.[5]

Highly satisfactory. Off went our women physicians to enlist, to join any of the Canadian medical teams, working with men or women, and by the end of the war, more than a hundred of them had served in the forces: 79 in the Royal Canadian Army Medical Corps, 14 in the Royal Canadian Air Force and 7 in the Royal Canadian Navy.[6]

As the years have passed, there have been fewer and fewer occasions when the Federation has been called upon to play such an active role. It hasn't been necessary — women and medicine have become comfortable partners. But it is still serving the function for which it was first formed: to be a society for medical women. And it is still useful in its secondary role too. It hasn't been active as a watchdog for some time now, but a watchdog doesn't have to growl in order to protect the house. Its presence is enough.

This presence is still needed, and possibly will always be needed, for although women physicians now officially have the same opportunities as male physicians, their situation isn't entirely equal — and it's doubtful if it ever will be. After all, males are males, and females are females. This is one of the facts of life and we live with its consequences, for legislation can't alter either character or characteristics. Too often, a woman has to be better than a man to fill a similar job; and certainly a mediocre woman can't get nearly as far as a mediocre man. She has to shine, and she also has to avoid being 'difficult'. One woman doctor's bad temper or incompetence can give the entire sex a bad name professionally.

This isn't as common as it used to be, but as late as 1936, Dr Helen Evans Reid had the greatest difficulty in being admitted to Toronto's Hospital for Sick Children, simply because there had been trouble with a previous woman resident there. The Physician-in-Chief had decided that women were a nuisance and that he wouldn't accept any more. Although Dr Reid was eventually admitted, it wasn't because of a change in policy. It was because of her own determination, because she launched a get-into-the-hospital campaign, sending off a stream of letters, telegrams and applications until the hospital couldn't stand it any longer. Very much in the tradition of earlier women doctors. But Helen Reid's campaign didn't take place in the 1880's. It went into action as late as 1936.

Naturally, prejudice against women in medicine didn't die a sudden death at the end of the First War. It was a gradual and continuing process, which is still going on today. All the same, the opportunities did increase very swiftly as a result of the war, and during the twenties and thirties women physicians found that they had far more scope than they had had in the first decade of the century. At last they were moving in relatively large numbers into the hospitals and universities, into truly general practice and into specialist fields. They were being given work that was mentally tough — and they were also being offered jobs that were tough physically. Female as well as male doctors were recruited to pioneer the North, Canada's last frontier.

When immigrant settlers moved into northern Alberta in the late 1920's the provincial government advertised for a group of lady doctors to take on some of the medical work, and four women were appointed. One of these was Dr Margaret Owens (Toronto, 1925), who was recruited to work in a travelling clinic, and the other three were from England.[7]

Dr Mary Percy Jackson was one of the English doctors, and the letters she wrote home to her family,[8] describe a practice that sounds very similar to that of Charlotte Ross at Whitemouth. But there was one important difference. Mary Percy was functioning on her own. This was a new generation of women doctors who didn't have the security of husband and family and weren't expected to need it. When Mary Percy arrived in Canada in 1929, Evelyn Windsor had recently started her work at Gleichen. Mary Percy's was the same type of work, except that she had no hospital or nurses, or even neighbours. She was taking on a really tough frontier practice, working alone and living alone — just as a male frontier doctor would do.

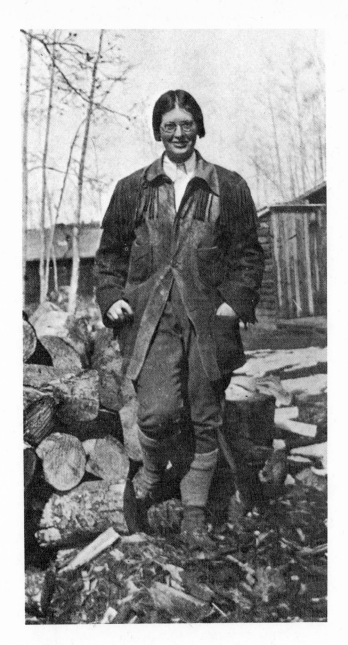

Dr Mary Percy Jackson at Peace River

She was sent to Battle River in the Peace River district, where she was provided with a small shack to act as house and surgery, and a horse to act as her transport. Mary was a city girl from Birmingham, England, but she was a keen horsewoman and one of the reasons why she had answered the provincial government's advertisement was that she was attracted by the idea of riding to her work. She had no experience of the Canadian climate, but she had experience in all the necessary areas — midwifery, surgery, anaesthetics, general practice — and she also had a great thirst for adventure. This was fortunate, because simply living in the Peace River district was an adventure.

It was in the first stage of settlement when Dr Percy arrived. The immigrants, many of them from middle Europe, were still moving in, and the community was both small and scattered. There was no other house within about half a mile, no telegraph, no road, and no bridge across the river — Dr Percy had to ford it to visit most of her patients. In winter she was sometimes snowed in for days on end (all alone in her small cabin) and when she was away on a case for more than a few hours, she would return to find her wood fire burnt out and everything frozen *inside* the house — the tea solid in the teapot, and the doorhandles and furniture so icy that she could get frostburns from touching them.

Her practice covered an area of about four hundred miles, the nearest hospital being a hundred miles away at Peace River. This meant that Dr Percy had to be surgeon as well as physician, for she couldn't send a patient to Peace River in midwinter — the journey could kill him. If he didn't die of shock, he might die of exposure. Later on, roads were built, cars and trucks could be used, and help could be cabled for by telegraph, but Dr Percy didn't enjoy these benefits for long. She moved on, farther north, to Keg River, for she had become Dr Percy Jackson, marrying a settler there.

Dr Percy Jackson is still at Keg River today. Like so many other women who came here from Europe, Canada became her country. Literally hundreds of immigrant women doctors have taken up work in Canada during the past fifty years — there are almost a thousand of them practising here today — and they represent a very powerful force in Canadian medicine. Like Mary Percy Jackson, they are doing the jobs which need to be done. Nowadays these jobs are seldom on the frontier. More often they are in high calibre laboratories in the hospitals and universities — one only needs to glance at the staff lists of almost any specialized research group to realize what a very important contribution our foreign-born and foreign-trained doctors are making. And of course they are not only working in specialist fields. In just about every branch of medicine, from general practice to neuroanatomy, you can find women physicians from Hungary, Germany, Britain, the United States, Poland, Russia, Scandinavia, Japan . . . from almost every country in the world. Including, of course, France.

The last quarter of a century has seen a great blossoming of women physicians in French Canada. It had been lack of opportunity, not lack of vocation, that had kept their numbers so small during the pioneering years, simply because there had been nowhere in Canada where they could study in their own language. Only a small minority were able to graduate as physicians — the few who could afford to travel to France, or those who spoke English so well that they could study at anglophone universities.

But this situation changed in the 1940's. Laval graduated its first woman MD in 1940. By that time, l'Université de Montreal was open to women. Since then, more than four hundred women have graduated from Canada's French-speaking universities and many of them are now playing a leading role in the field of medicine. It is a varied role, sometimes traditional and sometimes creating traditions. For instance, Dr Jeanne Lapierre (Montréal, 1950) is a medical missionary in Brazil — and, before she went there, she founded the Hôpital de la Visitation in Montreal. All very much in the tradition of her predecessors. But Dr Colette Perras (Montréal, 1948) is less traditional: she is head of plastic surgery at Montreal's Hôtel Dieu. And Dr Lise Fortier (Montréal, 1950), is both following and leading. As a champion of Women's Liberation, she can be linked with the many earlier women who were suffragettes — but of course there is a difference, for Dr Fortier doesn't have to fight for her position in medicine: she is a very prominent member of the profession. Perhaps the best known of all French Canada's medical women, Dr Fortier is President of the Planned Parenthood Federation of Canada, and gynaecologist and obstetrician at Notre Dame Hospital.

Each year the number of French-speaking medical women is growing — almost by compound interest — especially as there are now two more universities where they can study medicine: l'Université d'Ottawa and l'Université de Sherbrooke. Meanwhile, the women of English Canada have also been given more university places. In 1924, the University of Western Ontario graduated its first woman MD; in 1947, Queen's graduated the first women of its second experiment, and, in 1957, the University of Saskatchewan joined the ranks. The other universities accepted women as soon as their Faculties of Medicine were started, and in fact the first person to receive a medical degree from the University of Alberta was a woman, Dr Leone McGregor. Being the only girl in her class, she was gallantly called to the platform first. Nowadays there is seldom only one girl graduate in a class. In some universities there are as many as sixty. About two hundred women are graduating in medicine each year, and this is bringing the total of women physicians in Canada up to the four thousand mark.

With so many women in the profession, naturally a good proportion have made important contributions to medicine, and not only in recent years. There was Gladys Boyd for instance (Toronto, 1918), who became an internationally recognized authority on childhood nephritis and who was one of the first physicians in Canada to treat diabetic children with insulin. Lillian Chase (Toronto, 1922) was also well known for her work with insulin. Then there was Jessie Gray (Toronto, 1934), an outstanding surgeon and the only Canadian ever to be honoured with the Elizabeth Blackwell citation of the New York Infirmary. There was Ethlyn Trapp (McGill, 1927), a Canadian pioneer in radiation for the treatment of cancer. And, of course, there was Marion Hilliard (Toronto, 1927), the well-known and much-loved obstetrician and gynaecologist at the Women's College Hospital.

There have been so many significant Canadian medical women during the past fifty years that, in mentioning the names of a few, one inevitably omits others of equal standing, but the point is not *who* were the most outstanding, but *how many* achieved high positions in the profession. Considering that women have been a minority in the profession as a whole, they have made a very large contribution to Canadian medicine.

One factor which greatly helped them to do so was, of course, the Women's College Hospital. By the end of the First World War, the hospital could already offer residencies as well as a number of

specialist positions and, in 1935, when the present ten-storey building was opened on Grenville Street, a large percentage of our
medical women were associated with it. Most women either trained
or worked there, or both. By the end of the Second War, the Women's College Hospital had become one of the busiest in Toronto,
and it reached full maturity when, in the 1950's, it was recognized
as a teaching hospital by the University of Toronto — in 1956 for
Gynaecology and Obstetrics, in 1957 for Surgery, and in 1959 in
the Department of Medicine.

This was a great event in the life of the hospital, adding enormously to its prestige and usefulness, but it wasn't such a catalytic
event for women physicians in general. By this time, hospital experience, residencies and staff positions had been opened to them
throughout the nation. They were being widely accepted in the
profession as *physicians,* rather than as female physicians.

In more recent years, women have become so thoroughly inte-
grated into the medical profession that their sex has ceased to be an
important issue. How much this has been happening was sym-
bolized in 1973 when Dr Bette Stephenson was elected President of
the Canadian Medical Association — one of the most prestigious
appointments available to any physician in Canada. The fact that
Dr Stephenson was warmly and glamorously feminine and had six
children was completely immaterial. She had already served as
President of the Ontario Medical Association and her election to
the CMA presidency was therefore a natural development arising
from the contribution she had already made and from her very
obvious ability to tackle such a job successfully. So it wasn't in spite
of her sex that she was elected, or because of it, but *regardless* of it.
Women doctors have come a long way since Emily Stowe was first
refused admission to the University of Toronto.

They have come a long way and it is because of the many women
who have taken steps for them — sometimes intentionally, but often
unintentionally simply because of their work. It isn't only the
suffragettes who deserve our gratitude. Every woman doctor has
contributed something. Whether she was a general practitioner
quietly looking after women and children in a small provincial
town, or whether she was a worked-off-her-feet surgeon in a busy
city hospital; whether she was a pioneer gaining fame for her courage, or an academic gaining fame for her scholarship; whether she

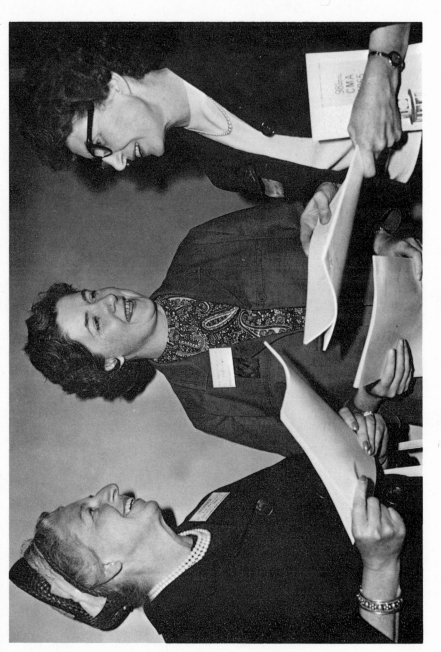

*Annual Meeting of the Federation of Medical Women of Canada, 1965
Left to right: Dr Eva Mader Macdonald, past President; Dr Bernice Russell Wylie, President;
Dr Maureen Roberts, incoming President*

hadn't really meant to become a doctor, but had done so because it would be useful; or whether she had always felt a driving urge to prove to the whole world that women could be physicians and very competent ones at that. . . . Whatever her calling — suffragette, missionary or war heroine, general practitioner, welfare worker or homemaker — every single woman who has ever graduated or practised in medicine has contributed something towards the acceptance of women as physicians, has made it that much easier for today's young school-leaver to get accepted into university, study without hassle, graduate in medicine and then move on to work in whatever field most appeals to her.

Today's women medical students don't need to know this. Nevertheless, they are the heirs of a very rich family, a family which has seldom been rich financially, but which has been rich in courage, integrity, faith, hope—and charity too. But, above all, in dedication.

FEDERATION FOUNDERS

HELEN MacMURCHY (Toronto, 1900 MB, 1901 MD)

Helen MacMurchy was the first President of the Federation. Born in Toronto in 1862, she was educated there and taught at the Toronto Collegiate Institute before studying medicine. An active public-health worker, especially in the field of women and children, she held the position of Chief of the Division of Child Welfare in the Federal Department of Health from 1920 to 1934. She was the author of many reports and booklets and was editor of the *Canadian Nurse* between 1905 and 1913. In 1934 she was created CBE. She died in Toronto in 1953.

MAUDE ELIZABETH SEYMOUR ABBOTT (Bishop's, 1894)

1897 LRCP & s Edinburgh.
1898 Licentiate Quebec Provincial Board.
1910 MD CM McGill (*honoris causa*).
1925 Licentiate State of Pennsylvania.
1931 Fellow of the Royal College of Physicians of Canada.
1935 Fellow of the Royal Society of Medicine, London.
1936 LL D McGill.

ELIZABETH BAGSHAW (Toronto, 1905)

In 1973, Dr Bagshaw was made a Member of the Order of Canada and she flew to Ottawa to receive the award in person. At the time she was 92 years old and was still practising medicine in Hamilton. Dr Bagshaw had started her practice in 1906, making her house calls in those days by horse and buggy or by bicycle. In the early 1930's she set up and ran the first birth-control clinic in Canada. During her long life she has received many honours for her work, and she has also had a school named after her in Hamilton.

JENNIE SMILLIE ROBERTSON (Toronto, 1909)

Jennie Smillie (Mrs Robertson) was born in Huron County and worked as a schoolteacher before studying medicine. She interned in Philadelphia and later returned there to be the assistant to one of the top women surgeons at the women's hospital. Dr Smillie's main interest was surgery and she was one of the first women to practise surgery in Canada, and the first to perform major surgery at the Women's College Hospital. She also specialized in gynaecology. She married at the age of 70.

ELIZABETH EMBURY (Queen's, 1888)
Elizabeth Embury was one of Canada's very early women graduates and she
practised in Belleville until 1906 when she moved to Ottawa. She died in 1945.

JANET HALL (Trinity, 1899)
Dr Hall did postgraduate work in Europe and then returned to her home town
of Woodstock to open a general practice. She worked there until four years
before her death in 1950.

SOME PAST PRESIDENTS OF THE FEDERATION OF
MEDICAL WOMEN OF CANADA

GLADYS BOYD (Toronto, 1918. President of the Federation 1932-33)
From 1921 to 1950, Dr Boyd headed the Endocrine Service at the Hospital for
Sick Children in Toronto and she was one of the first physicians to treat
diabetic children with insulin. As Associate Professor in Paediatrics at the
University of Toronto and as a member of the medical research staff of the
Hospital for Sick Children, she directed research and treatment in diabetes,
nephritis and tuberculosis, and she became an internationally recognized
authority on childhood nephritis. She died in 1970.

ETHLYN TRAPP (McGill, 1927. President of the Federation 1946-47)
In 1968 Dr Trapp was awarded the medal of service of the Order of Canada.
She was one of the first physicians in Canada to use radiotherapy in the
treatment of cancer, and during the Second World War she was Acting Director
of the British Columbia Cancer Institute. After the war, she was elected
President of the B.C. Medical Association and in 1952-53 she was made
President of the National Cancer Institute of Canada. She was the first woman
to hold either position. Dr Trapp died in Vancouver in 1972.

MARGARET OWENS (Toronto, 1925. President of the Federation 1947-48)
From 1927 to 1935, Dr Owens worked as a member of Alberta's travelling clinic.
The clinic was a public health service, supported by the provincial government, and it consisted of a small group of doctors, dentists and nurses who
travelled the province — sometimes doing as much as 8000 miles a year —
examining the rural communities. In 1937 Dr Owens settled in Winnipeg,
where one of her concerns was birth control.

MARY ANNA NICHOLSON WRIGHT (Toronto, 1925. President of the
Federation 1949-50)
Dr Nicholson (Mrs Wright) was an anaesthetist. Born in Ontario, she settled
in Saskatoon where she was on the staff of the City Hospital and St Paul's
Hospital.

JESSIE McGEACHY MACLEOD (Toronto, 1937. President of the
Federation 1959-60)
Jessie McGeachy (Mrs Macleod) was a nurse before she became a doctor. As a
physician, she worked in Toronto, Halifax, Winnipeg, Saskatoon and Ottawa

and when she died in 1966 she was staff physician in the psychiatric unit at the Royal Ottawa Sanitarium and Lecturer at the University of Ottawa.

EMMA RICHTER ADAMSON (Manitoba, 1929. President of the Federation 1962-63)
Emma Adamson ran a general practice in Winnipeg, with the emphasis on psychosomatic medicine and psychiatry.

ENID JOHNSON MacLEOD (Dalhousie, 1937. President of the Federation 1969-70)
Enid Johnson (Mrs MacLeod) was born in Jacksonville, N.B., and her early education was in New Brunswick and Nova Scotia. The daughter of a minister, she had originally intended to be a medical missionary, but after her graduation she decided to stay in Canada. In 1939 Enid Johnson met Dr H.R. Griffith who asked her to work with him in anaesthesia, so she studied anaesthesia for three years and became a certified specialist in the subject. With Dr Griffith, she pioneered the use of curare as a muscle relaxant, and she gave the first anaesthetic in which Dr Griffith used curare for this purpose. In 1942 Enid Johnson married Innis G. MacLeod and for six years she practised anaesthesia in Sydney, Nova Scotia. In 1960 she joined the Physiology Department of Dalhousie Medical School, where she now holds the position of Associate Professor.

FIVE NON-CANADIAN GRADUATES

MARY PERCY JACKSON (Birmingham, 1927)

Mary Percy won the Queen's prize when she graduated from Birmingham
University — holding the highest aggregate marks in medicine, surgery and
midwifery. After interning in medicine, obstetrics and anaesthetics, and
working as a house surgeon at the Children's Hospital in Birmingham,
where she gained experience in minor surgery, she came to Canada
in 1929 and for two years served as frontier doctor at Battle River
in the Peace River district. In 1931, she married Frank Jackson and moved
further north to Keg River, where she intended to be a pioneer wife rather
than a doctor. But she was the only qualified physician within several hundred
miles, so once again she found herself ministering to the isolated settlers and
the many Métis of the district. Dr Percy Jackson continued to practise in the
north, while bringing up a family, helping with the family farm, serving as
school trustee and continually pressing for improved conditions for the Métis.

EMMA MARY JOHNSTONE (Edinburgh, 1910)

Dr Johnstone worked in mental hospitals in Great Britain before she came
to Canada in 1927. She then became a country district doctor in Alberta, and
it was she who wrote the provincial government's advertisement which
brought Dr Percy Jackson to Canada. During the Second World War,
Dr Johnstone returned to England and served so gallantly during the air raids
that she was awarded the OBE. After the war, she came back to Canada and
worked in northern Alberta until her retirement.

MARIA ZUROWSKA (Lwow, 1930)

Born in Poland in 1901, Dr Zurowska specialized in tuberculosis at the Lwow
University Institute of Hygiene and Bacteriology until 1941. From 1944 to
1948 she served as a paediatrician in Gdansk, Poland, and then spent two
years working in a Displaced Persons camp in Germany. She immigrated to
Canada in 1950 and took up general practice at Moose Factory, Windsor,
London and Sudbury. In 1967 she was awarded the Centennial Medal.

MARGARET BEZNAK (Budapest, 1939)

Born and educated in Hungary, Dr Beznak was an assistant professor at
Birmingham University, England, before she came to Canada. A specialist
in physiology, she has written about 60 scientific papers, most of them on
cardiovascular physiology. She joined the staff of the University of Ottawa

in 1953. Since then, she has been appointed Head of the Department of
Physiology, Vice-Dean of Medicine and a member of the university's Board of
Governors. In 1964 Dr Beznak was named first winner of the University of
Ottawa Dow Brewery Staff Research Lectureship, an award given annually to
a member of the university staff whose work is of exceptional distinction.

SHEILA MAUREEN McWILLIAM ROBERTS (Edinburgh, 1937)
Maureen McWilliam (Mrs Roberts) was born in Peterhead, Scotland, and she
came to Canada in 1948, having previously worked in hospitals in England
and having served in the Indian Medical Service during the Second World War.
In Canada, Dr Roberts worked first in Halifax, both in the hospitals and as
Assistant Professor of Paediatrics at Dalhousie where, at the newly established
chromosome laboratory, she conducted chromosomal investigations on patients
in the children's hospital. In 1964-65 she was one of the two women doctors
who took part in the Canadian Medical Expedition to Easter Island — the
other being Dr HELEN EVANS REID (Alberta, 1935). In 1965 Dr Roberts
moved to Ottawa where she organized the chromosome laboratory at the
University of Ottawa and where she became Associate Professor of Paediatrics
at the University of Ottawa and Consultant in Paediatrics (genetics) at
Ottawa General Hospital. She was President of the Federation of Medical
Women of Canada 1965-66.

QUEBECKERS

LISE FORTIER (Montreal, 1950)

Dr Fortier was born and educated in Montreal and graduated from the Université de Montréal in 1950. She specialized in obstetrics and gynaecology, joining the staff of Notre Dame Hospital and the Université de Montréal, where she is Assistant Professor in Obstetrics and Gynaecology. Dr Fortier holds strong views on a woman's right to have control over her own body and feels that abortions should not be governed by laws. She has always been active in the field of family planning and holds the position of President of the Planned Parenthood Federation of Canada.

EVA ARENDT RACINE (McGill, 1949)

Eva Arendt (Mrs Racine) was born in China. She interned at the Queen Elizabeth Hospital and did her residency at the Montreal General. She then served on the staff of the Montreal General where she was appointed Director of the Nurses Health Service. She specialized in rheumatology and is Consultant in Rheumatology at the Queen Mary Veteran's Hospital and at the Reddy Memorial Hospital. Dr Arendt Racine is also Assistant Professor of Medicine at McGill University. In 1961-62 she was President of the Federation of Medical Women of Canada.

BLANDINE GOSSELIN (Montreal, 1951)

Dr Gosselin was born in Manitoba and her family moved to Quebec when she was seven years old. After graduating from Montreal, she worked as a resident in hospitals in Montreal and New York until 1957, when she joined the staff of Notre Dame Hospital, Montreal. Since 1966, she has been head of the Service d'Hématologie at Notre Dame Hospital.

ANTONINE PAQUIN (Montreal, 1954)

Dr Paquin is head of the Health Department, City of Montreal.

THERESE DESCHENES-CARTIER (Montreal, 1949)

Dr Deschênes-Cartier is an anaesthetist at Hôtel Dieu, Montreal.

COLETTE PERRAS (Montreal, 1948)

Dr Perras is head of the plastic surgery department at Hôtel Dieu Hospital.

CLAUDE-LISE RICHER (Montreal, 1954)

Dr Richer is professor in the Faculty of Medicine at the Université de Montréal and Vice-Dean in charge of postgraduate studies.

GEORGETTE GELINAS (Laval, 1943)
Dr Gélinas is a paediatrician and Director of Public Health at Ville St Laurent.

CLAIRE GELINAS-MACKAY (Montreal, 1943)
Claire Gélinas (Mrs Mackay) was born in Grand'Mère, Quebec, and was
educated in Trois-Rivières, Ottawa and Montreal before attending the
Université de Montréal. After graduation, she specialized in pathology and
she is now pathologist at Notre Dame Hospital and Assistant Professor of
Pathology at the Université de Montréal.

SOME POST-WAR GRADUATES ASSOCIATED WITH
THE WOMEN'S COLLEGE HOSPITAL

JESSIE GRAY (Toronto, 1934)

In 1954, Dr Jessie Gray received the Elizabeth Blackwell Award of the
New York Infirmary and was named the leading woman surgeon in Canada.
At the time, she was Chief of Surgery at the Women's College Hospital. She
attained many 'firsts' in surgery: first woman to take the Gallie course in
surgery, first woman resident surgeon at Toronto General Hospital, first
woman to become a Fellow of the Royal College of Surgeons of Canada and
first woman to be a member of the Central Surgical Society of North America.

MARION GRANT KERR (Toronto, 1919)

Dr Kerr served as Chief of Obstetrics and Gynaecology at the Women's College
Hospital from 1926 to 1947. After retirement she was an active consultant to
the hospital. She died in 1951.

ANNA MARION HILLIARD (Toronto, 1927)

Born in Morrisburg, Ontario, in 1902, Marion Hilliard joined the staff of the
Women's College Hospital in 1928. She specialized in obstetrics and
gynaecology, building up a large obstetrical practice, and acting as friend
and counsellor as well as physician to her many patients. Dr Hilliard
succeeded Marion Kerr as Chief of Service in Obstetrics and Gynaecology and
she was largely responsible for establishing the Cancer Detection Clinic
associated with the hospital. By her work and her outgoing personality, she
enormously increased the prestige of the Women's College Hospital, and it
was while she was Chief of Obstetrics and Gynaecology that the department
was accorded teaching status by the University of Toronto. In 1955-56
Marion Hilliard was President of the Federation of Medical Women of Canada.
She died in 1958 at the age of 56.

FLORENCE HARDY McCONNEY (Toronto, 1920)

Florence Hardy (Mrs McConney) was born in Lindsay, Ontario, and she was
associated with the Women's College Hospital for 50 years. For 15 of those
years, she held the position of Chief of Medicine, and for 10 she was Director
of the Cancer Detection Clinic.

JEAN DAVEY (Toronto, 1936)

In 1950 Jean Davey succeeded Florence McConney as Chief of Medicine at
the Women's College Hospital. She was born in Hamilton, Ontario, and after

graduation she interned at the Toronto General Hospital and the Women's College Hospital. During the Second World War, Dr Davey held the position of Squadron Leader in the RCAF where she was responsible for the medical aspects of the Women's Division. In 1943 she was awarded the OBE and in 1973 she was created an Officer of the Order of Canada. She was on the staff of the University of Toronto from 1956 to 1973, rising to the position of Professor in the Faculty of Medicine.

ELLEN COMISKY BLATCHFORD (Toronto, 1923)

Ellen Comisky (Mrs Blatchford) went to high school in Aurora before registering as a student at the University of Toronto. She joined the staff of the Women's College Hospital as an anaesthetist and in 1932 she was appointed Chief of the Department of Anaesthesia. She held this position until 1955, when she became an active consultant. Dr Blatchford retired in 1967.

HENRIETTA BANTING (Toronto, 1945)

Lady Banting, the wife of Sir Frederick Banting, entered the University of Toronto as a medical student a few months after her husband was killed on active service. On graduation, she served with the Royal Canadian Army Medical Corps and then took postgraduate training in England and taught at the University Medical School in Hong Kong before returning to Canada to join the staff of the Women's College Hospital. She was appointed Director of the hospital's Cancer Detection Clinic and she specialized in this field until she retired. For eight years, she served as the Vice-President of the Medical Women's International Association.

NOTES

CHAPTER 1

1 Dr Barry's full name is given in her own handwriting on the flyleaf of her copy of *Orations of Cicero,* which is now in the library of the Royal Army Medical College, London, England.
2 Isobel Rae, *The Strange Story of Dr James Barry* (London, Longmans, 1958).
3 George Thomas Keppel, Earl of Albemarle, *Fifty Years of my Life* (London, 1876), Vol. 2, p. 96.
4 Isobel Rae, *op. cit.*
5 Public Record Office, London, *Roll of Commissioned Officers in Medical Service in the Army.*
Harts Army List, 1864.
6 Isobel Rae, *op. cit.*
7 Personal communication from Isobel Rae.
8 Memorandum by Dr Barry, Public Record Office, London, WO.138/1.
9 *Encyclopaedia Britannica,* 11th ed. (1910), Vol. 3, pp. 444-445.
10 Miranda papers.
11 P.R. Kirby, 'Dr James Barry, Controversial South African Medical Figure: A Recent Evaluation of his Life and Sex,' *South African Medical Journal* (April 25, 1970), pp. 506-516.

CHAPTER 2

1 Joanne Emily Thompson, *The Influence of Dr Emily Howard Stowe on the Woman Suffrage Movement in Canada,* Unpublished thesis, the University College of Waterloo Lutheran University, 1962, Wilfrid Laurier University.
2 F.C. Gullen, *Gullen History,* Manuscript scrapbook of Stowe, Lossing and Gullen families, Archives, Victoria University, Toronto.

3 Personal information from Mr Hudson Stowe.
4 Manuscript document by Dr Emily Stowe, Morgan Collection, Public Archives of Canada, Ottawa.
5 F.C. Gullen, *op. cit.*
6 N. Burwash, *History of Victoria College* (Toronto, Victoria College Press, c. 1927).
7 This college was founded in 1863 by Dr Clemence Sophia Lozier, and in 1866 it changed its name to the New York Medical College and Hospital for Women, Homeopathic (cf. J.J. Walsh, *History of Medicine in New York,* 1919 and *American Medical Directory,* 1923). It should not be confused with the Woman's Medical College of the New York Infirmary for Women and Children (which was established by Elizabeth Blackwell and her sister, Emily, and graduated its first class in 1870).
8 Emily Stowe graduated in 1867 (cf. The *Sixth Annual Announcement* of the New York Medical College for Women). She was established in Toronto and advertising for patients in 1867 (cf. *The Globe,* Nov. 11, 1867; Dec. 3, 1867, etc.).
9 *Ontario Medical Act,* 32 Victoria, Cap. XLV.
10 *Annual Announcement* of the Toronto School of Medicine, 1869-70, University of Toronto Archives.
11 Newspaper cutting in *Scrapbook No. 4,* Stowe Collection, Wilfrid Laurier University Archives.
12 Newspaper cutting in *Scrapbook No. 3,* Stowe Collection, Wilfrid Laurier University Archives.
13 Elizabeth Smith-Shortt, 'Historical Sketch of Medical Education of Women in Kingston,' Paper read before the Osler Club, Queen's University, Sept. 14, 1916.
14 Elizabeth Stanton, Susan B. Anthony and Matilda J. Gage, eds., *History of Woman Suffrage* (Rochester, Charles Man, 1887). Hilda Ridley, *A Synopsis of Woman Suffrage in Canada,* Undated booklet, Stowe Collection, Victoria University Archives.
15 Newspaper Cuttings, Stowe Scrapbooks, Stowe Collection, Wilfrid Laurier University Archives.
16 *Ibid.*
17 *Ibid.*
18 The Pavilion was built in 1878, in what is now known as Allan Gardens. It was used as a concert hall and for dramatic performances as well as flower displays. It burnt down in 1902.
19 *Toronto City Directories,* 1867-1878.
20 F.C. Gullen, *op. cit.*
21 Manuscript Document by Dr Emily Stowe, *op. cit.*
22 F.C. Gullen, *op. cit.*
23 Manuscript Document by Dr Emily Stowe, *op. cit.*
24 Newspaper cutting in *Scrapbook No. 3, op. cit.*
25 *The Globe* (Toronto), May 18, 1883.
26 Personal information from Miss Hilda I. Stowe.
27 *The British Whig* (Kingston), Jan. 6, 1883.

28 Augusta Stowe-Gullen, *A Brief History of the Ontario Medical College for Women,* 1906.
29 *The Globe* (Toronto), Dec. 4, 1928.
30 *Globe and Mail* (Toronto), Sept. 27, 1943.
31 *Mail and Empire* (Toronto), Oct. 24, 1928.
32 F.C. Gullen, *op. cit.*
33 Personal communication from Miss Hilda I. Stowe.

CHAPTER 3

1 W.H. Trout, *Trout Family History* (Milwaukee, Meyer-Rotier Printing Co., 1916), p. 280.
2 *Ibid.,* p. 281.
3 Article on 'Woman Suffrage in Canada' in Stowe *Scrapbook No. 3,* Stowe Collection, Wilfrid Laurier University Archives.
4 W.H. Trout, *op. cit.*
5 *Toronto City Directories,* 1866-1873. The Stowes lived at 135 Church Street before they bought the house at 111 Church Street in 1878.
6 Material on the Gowanlock family in the Stratford area was provided by Mr James Anderson, Archivist, Perth County Archives.
7 Henry James Morgan, ed., *The Canadian Men and Women of the Time,* 2nd ed. (Toronto, William Briggs, 1912), p. 1110.
8 W.H. Trout, *op. cit.,* p. 275.
9 Diary of Elizabeth Smith, April 24, 1879, Adam Shortt Papers, Queen's University Archives.
10 Student lists, Alumnae, Woman's Medical College of Pennsylvania.
11 W.H. Trout, *op. cit.* pp. 280-281.
12 *The Globe* (Toronto), July 24, 1875.
13 *Toronto City Directory,* 1877.
14 Diary of Elizabeth Smith, *op. cit.*
15 W.H. Trout, *op. cit.,* p. 281.
16 David Edwards, 'Mrs Jenny K. Trout, MD,' *Notabilities of Toronto,* No. 1, for subscribers only, 50¢., Perth County Archives (Toronto, Peter A. Gross, 1877).
17 Elizabeth Smith-Shortt, 'Historical Sketch of Medical Education of Women in Kingston', Paper read before the Osler Club, Queen's University, Sept. 14, 1916.
18 *Ibid.*
19 Henry James Morgan, *op. cit.*
20 *Annual Calendar of the Kingston Women's Medical College in Affiliation with Queen's University,* 1886-87, Queen's University Archives.
21 W.H. Trout, *op. cit.*

CHAPTER 4

1 Diary of Elizabeth Smith, April 23, 1879, Adam Shortt Papers, Queen's University Archives.

2 Elizabeth Smith-Shortt, Typescript biography, Adam Shortt Papers, Queen's University Archives.
3 Diary of Elizabeth Smith, *op. cit.*
4 Adam Shortt Papers, Queen's University Archives.
5 *Ibid.*
6 *Ibid.*
7 Letter of Elizabeth Smith, May 20, 1880, Adam Shortt Papers, Queen's University Archives.
8 *Queen's College Journal,* Vol. 3, No. 1 (Kingston, October 30, 1880).
9 Letter of Elizabeth Smith, October 20, 1881, Adam Shortt Papers, Queen's University Archives.
10 *Ibid.,* 1882.
11 Diary of Elizabeth Smith, 1882, *op. cit.*
12 *Ibid.,* April, 1882.
13 *Weekly Globe* (Toronto), December 22, 1882.
14 Annual Announcements of Kingston Women's Medical College, Queen's University Archives.
15 *Ibid.*
16 Charlotte Whitton, 'An Appreciation of Mrs Adam Shortt,' *Queen's College Journal* (Feb. 1949), pp. 39-41.
17 *Canadian Medical Association Journal,* Obituary, Vol. 2, No. 12 (December, 1912), p. 1150.
18 Jean Sinclair MacKay, 'Elizabeth Beatty, MD,' *The Missionary Monthly* (May, 1940), pp. 207-208.

CHAPTER 5

1 *Morning Herald* (Halifax), August 13, 1883.
2 Information from Dean's Office, Dalhousie University.
3 *Belcher's Farmer's Almanack,* 1880-1900, Medical Registers.
4 *Liverpool Advance* (Liverpool, Nova Scotia), April 27, 1898.
5 *Saint John Globe* (Saint John, New Brunswick), July 6, 1916.
6 Personal communication from Dr Secord's nephew, Clarence B. Smith.
7 The basic information on Dr Ross is drawn from personal communication with her granddaughter, Mrs E.A. Backman, and from papers in the Provincial Archives of Manitoba.
8 Birth Certificate, Somerset House, London.
9 Pierre Berton, *The National Dream* (Toronto, McClelland and Stewart, 1970), pp. 245-247.
10 Student lists, Alumnae, Woman's Medical College of Pennsylvania.
11 *Mackay's Montreal Directory,* 1876-1877.
12 *Winnipeg Street Directory,* 1912 and 1913.
13 *Calgary Daily Herald,* April 23, 1913.
14 *Alumni Catalog,* Michigan Historical Collection, the University of Michigan.
15 *The Manitoba Medical Register,* Register No. 2, College of Physicians and Surgeons of Manitoba, Winnipeg.

16 *Winnipeg Free Press,* September 22, 1882.
17 Undated newspaper clipping in Stowe Scrapbooks, Stowe Collection, Wilfrid Laurier University.
18 *Winnipeg Free Press,* March 25, 1901.
19 E. Cora Hind, 'Dr Amelia Yeomans', *Manitoba Messenger,* June 1913, p. 9.
20 James H. Gray, *Red Lights on the Prairies* (Toronto, The Macmillan Company of Canada, 1971).
21 E. Cora Hind, *op. cit.*
22 *Winnipeg Free Press,* April 28, 1899.
23 *Calgary Daily Herald,* April 23, 1913.
24 Street Directories of Winnipeg and Calgary.
25 United Church Archives, Toronto.

CHAPTER 6

1 Dorothy Middleton, *Victorian Lady Travellers* (London, Routledge & Kegan Paul, Ltd., 1965), pp. 107-127
2 *The Christian Guardian,* June 12, 1901.
3 Adam Shortt Papers, Queen's University Archives.
4 *Annual Calendar,* 1905, Ontario Medical College for Women. List of graduates.
5 The story of the Rijnharts' mission to Tibet is drawn from: Dr Susie C. Rijnhart, *With the Tibetans in Tent and Temple* (Fleming H. Revell Co., 1901).
6 *Ibid.,* p. 111.
7 Sven Hedin, *Through Asia,* Vol. 2 (London, Methuen & Co., 1898), p. 1173.
8 Student Cards, University of Toronto Records Office.
9 The Methodist Church of Canada, *Our West China Mission,* Toronto 1920.
10 Esther Pohl Lovejoy, *Women Doctors of the World* (New York, The Macmillan Company, 1957), p. 233.
11 Dr Susie C. Rijnhart, *op. cit.*
12 Pat Barr, *To China with Love* (London, Secker and Warburg, 1972), p. 194.
13 United Church Archives, Toronto.
14 Details of Dr Chute's life from personal information provided by her son, Dr A.L. Chute and her daughter, Miss L. Chute.
15 Rev. M.L. Orchard and Miss K.S. McLaurin, *The Enterprise,* The Jubilee Story of the Canadian Baptist Mission in India, 1874-1924 (The Canadian Baptist Foreign Mission Board, Toronto, 1924).
16 Flora Clarke, *Sisters: Canada and India* (Moncton, N.B., Maritime Press, 1939).

CHAPTER 7

1 Material on Dr Matheson is from personal information provided by her daughter, Ruth Matheson Buck, and from the following articles and talks by Ruth Matheson Buck:

'Unusual Parents,' Lecture to University Women's Club, Regina, 1952.

'The Mathesons of Saskatchewan Diocese' in *Saskatchewan History,* Vol. XIII, 1960.

Address to Mother's Union, St Paul's Pro-Cathedral, 1961.

'Making of a Doctor', *Century 1867/1967,* Southam Press, February 13, 1967.

'The Mathesons of Onion Lake', *Homestead Memories,* 1967.

2 University of Manitoba *Calendars* for 1891-93.

3 The North-West Territories of Canada *Medical Register,* 1894. Canadian Medical Association, Edmonton.

4 Helen Evans Reid, *All Silent, All Damned* (Toronto, Ryerson Press, 1969).

5 *Canadian Medical Association Journal,* Vol. 3, No. 2 (February, 1913), p. 116.

6 *Canadian Medical Association Journal,* Obituary, Vol. 69, No. 6 (December, 1953), p. 651.

7 'History of the Canadian Nurse' in *Canadian Nurse,* Vol. 5, No. 3 (March, 1909), pp. 193-197.

8 *Canadian Medical Association Journal,* Vol. 10, No. 7 (July 1920), p. 681.

9 'Dr Eliza Perley Brison' in *The Social Welfare Pioneers in Nova Scotia,* No. 3 (1972).

10 Personal information from Miss Lillian Romkey.

11 H.E. MacDermot, *One Hundred Years of Medicine in Canada* (Toronto, McClelland and Stewart, 1967), p. 16.

CHAPTER 8

1 Personal communication from Dr Jacques Abourbih.

2 The basic information on Dr Abbott has been drawn from:
   Maude E. Abbott, 'Autobiographical Sketch,' 1928, printed in *McGill Medical Journal* 28: 127-152, Montreal, 1959.
   H.E. MacDermot, *Maude Abbott: A Memoir* (Toronto, The Macmillan Company of Canada, 1941).
   Jessie Boyd Scriver, 'Maude E. Abbott' in Mary Quayle Innis, ed., *The Clear Spirit* (Toronto, University of Toronto Press, 1966), Chap. 8.
   and from papers in the Archives of the Osler Library, McGill University.

3 Maude E. Abbott, *op. cit.*

4 Jacques Abourbih, 'FemLib Flashback' in *McGill Medical Journal,* Vol. 40, 1971.

5 H.E. MacDermot, *op. cit.,* p. 36.

6 *Ibid.,* pp. 41-42.

7 E.H. Bensley, 'Bishop's Medical College' in *Canadian Medical Association Journal* Vol. 72, No. 6 (March 15, 1955), pp. 463-465.

8 Maude E. Abbott, *op. cit.,* p. 152.

9 *Ibid.,* p. 146.

10 *Canadian Medical Association Journal,* Vol. 8, No. 7 (July, 1918), p. 657.

11 Jessie Boyd Scriver, 'McGill's First Women Medical Students' in *McGill Medical Journal* (1947), pp. 237-243.
12 *Canadian Medical Association Journal*, Vol. 8, No. 6 (June, 1918), p. 554.
13 H.E. MacDermot, *op. cit.*, p. 198.

CHAPTER 9

1 Elizabeth L. Stewart, *A Brief History of the Women's College Hospital*, 1956.
2 Ontario Medical College for Women, *Annual Calendar*, 1905.
3 Albiny Paquette, 'Irma LeVasseur (1877-1964)' in souvenir booklet printed to celebrate 40th anniversary of L'Hôpital de l'Enfant-Jésus (1963), pp. 61-62.
4 *La Patrie* (Montreal), July 9, 1950.
5 *Gazette* (Montreal), June 22, 1950.
6 Albiny Paquette, *op. cit.*
7 *Encyclopaedia Britannica*, 12th ed., Vol. 32, p. 406.
8 *Canadian Medical Association Journal*, Vol. 5, No. 8 (August, 1915), p. 723; *CMAJ*, Vol. 5, No. 11 (November, 1915), p. 1028.
9 Esther Pohl Lovejoy, 'Women Doctors in World War I' in *Women Doctors of the World* (New York, The Macmillan Company, 1957), Chap. 20, pp. 277-307.
10 *Encyclopaedia Britannica*, 12th ed. (1922), Vol. 32, p. 1058.
11 Personal communication from Dr Edward.
12 Mary Lee Edward, Personal diary.
13 *Canadian Medical Association Journal*, Vol. 6, No. 11 (November, 1916), p. 1035.
14 Personal information provided by Dr Windsor's daughter, Mrs Joan Fellows.

CHAPTER 10

1 Details of Dr Windsor's life from personal information provided by her daughter, Mrs Joan Fellows, and her son, Mr Peter Leacock.
2 *Calgary Herald*, October 19, 1966, and *Canadian Medical Association Journal*, Vol. 61, No. 2 (August, 1949), p. 194.
3 *Canadian Medical Association Journal*, Vol. 8, No. 2 (February, 1918), p. 174.
4 Canon John House, *Old Sun Anglican Residential School, Gleichen, Alberta*. Glenbow-Alberta Institute, Calgary, 1933.
5 G.H. Gooderham, *Doctors to the Indians Whom I Have Known*, Typescript, Archives of Glenbow-Alberta Institute, Calgary, 1960.
6 Personal communication from Mr S.W. Horrall, Historian, RCMP, Ottawa.
7 *Leader Post, Regina*, (January 24, 1959).
RCMP Quarterly, Vol. 24, No. 4, (April, 1959).

8 Personal information on Dr McGill provided by S/Sgt. Major J. Robinson (retd.) who worked with her for many years.
9 *RCMP Quarterly,* Vol. 38, No. 3, (July, 1972).
10 *RCMP Quarterly,* Vol. 12, No. 1, January, 1946, and Ruth Matheson Buck, *Dr Frances McGill,* M.S.
11 Personal communication from Mr J.S. Dornan, Lands and Surveys Branch, Department of Natural Resources, Province of Saskatchewan.

CHAPTER 11

1 Federation of Medical Women of Canada, *Original Constitution,* 1925, Federation Archives, Ottawa.
2 Medical Women's International Association, *Bulletin,* No. 24, August, 1970.
3 Federation of Medical Women of Canada, *Minutes of Organizing Meeting,* 1924, Federation Archives, Ottawa.
4 *Minutes, op. cit.,* 1925.
5 *Ibid.,* 1942.
6 Dr Edna Guest, 'Report of War Services Committee', in Federation of Medical Women of Canada, *Minutes,* 1948, Federation Archives, Ottawa.
7 *Calgary Herald,* June 22, 1929.
8 Letters of Mary Percy Jackson, *On the Last Frontier* (London, The Sheldon Press; Toronto, General Board of Religious Education, 1933).

APPENDIX I

Women Graduates of Canada's Medical Colleges 1883-1895

1883
Augusta Stowe-Gullen (née Stowe) MD Victoria (via Toronto School of Medicine)

WOMEN'S MEDICAL COLLEGE *Kingston*	WOMAN'S MEDICAL COLLEGE *Toronto*	OTHER
1884 Elizabeth Beatty *Queen's* Alice McGillivray *Queen's* Elizabeth Smith-Shortt *Queen's* (née Smith)		
1885 Margaret Corliss *Queen's* Helen Ryan *Queen's* (née Reynolds)		
1886 Annie Dickson *Queen's* Marion Oliver *Queen's*		
1887 Ella Atherton *Queen's* (née Blaylock) Ada Funnell *Queen's* Marion Livingstone *Queen's*	Alice Constantineau *Trinity* (née McLaughlin) Annie Pickering *Trinity*	
1888 Agnes Craine *Queen's* Elizabeth Embury *Queen's* Annie Lawyer *Queen's* Elizabeth Mitchell *Queen's* Nettie Oughten *Queen's* (née Ogilvie)	Mary Buchanan *Trinity* (née McKay) Emma Jones *Trinity* (née Stone) Susanna Rijnhart *Trinity* (née Carson)	
1889 Isobel McConville *Queen's*	Jennie Carson *Trinity* Lelia Davis *Toronto* Stella Taylor *Trinity*	

1890
Sara Brown *Queen's*
Clara Demorest *Queen's*
Rose Funnell *Queen's*
Margaret MacKellar *Queen's*
Wilhelmina Stuart *Queen's*
(née Fraser)
Hattie Walker *Queen's*

Mary Agar *Trinity*
Susanna Hamilton *Trinity*
(née Boyle)
Ida Lynd *Trinity*
Mary McDonnell *Trinity*
(née Hutton)
Emily Smith *Toronto*
(née Irvine)

1891
Janet Murray *Queen's*
Margaret O'Hara *Queen's*
Janet Weir *Queen's*

Lucinda Graham *Trinity*
Alfretta Kilborn *Trinity*
(née Gifford)
Letitia Sirrs *Trinity*
(née Meade)
Julia Thomas *Trinity*

Grace Ritchie-England
(née Ritchie) *Bishop's*

1892
Elizabeth Henderson *Queen's*
Annie Hill *Queen's*
Alison Jamieson *Queen's*
Mary Macarow *Queen's*
(née Bermingham)
Nellie Skimmen *Queen's*
Agnes Turnbull *Queen's*

Annie Cleland *Trinity*
(née Chambers)
Harrietta Denovan *Victoria*
(née Paterson)
Bertha Dymond *Trinity*
Eliza Gray *Trinity*
Matilda Hill *Toronto*
(née Foster)
Eleanore Lennox *Ohio*
Jennie Wildman *Trinity*
(née Gray)

Harriet Clarke *Manitoba*
(née Foxton)

1893
Minnie Greer *Queen's*
(née Leavitt)
Clara Ryan *Queen's*

Minnie Campbell *Trinity*
(née Brander)
Eva Fisher *Trinity*
(née Ryan)
Annie Higbee *Trinity &*
Toronto (née Carveth)
Ellen Sherratt *Trinity*
(née Burt)

1894

Jennie Bloomfield *Trinity*
(née Shirra)
Nancy Chenoweth *Trinity*
(née Rodger)
Margaret Fleming *Trinity*
Gertrude Hulet *Trinity*
Marjorie Ward *Trinity*

Maude Abbott
Bishop's
Annie Hamilton
Dalhousie

1895
Jennie Drennan *Queen's*

Annie Alguire *Trinity*
(née McCallum)
Pearl Chute *Trinity*
(née Smith)
Mary Davidson *Trinity*
(née Allen)
Jeannie Dow *Toronto*
Margaret Forster *Trinity*
(née MacMillan)
Elizabeth Hurdon *Trinity*
Daisy Macklin *Trinity*
Jennie Mitchell *Trinity*
(née Hill)
Rose Pringle *Trinity*
Marguerite Symington
Trinity

Edythe Clendenning *Bishop's*
Josephine Cunin *Bishop's*
Regina Lewis-Landau *Bishop's*
Katherine Mackenzie
(née MacKay)
Dalhousie

NOTE: *Maiden names have not been given for women who graduated in their married names*

APPENDIX II
Women Graduates of Canada's Medical Colleges 1896-1905

ONTARIO MEDICAL COLLEGE FOR WOMEN	OTHER

1896
Emma Gordon *Toronto*
(née Skinner)
Annie Jones *Trinity*
(née Verth)
Christina Macklin *Toronto*
(née Sinclair)
Mary Rutnam *Trinity*
(née Irwin)
Tina Patrick *Trinity*
(née Head)

Mary Fyffe *Bishop's*
Clara Hebb *Dalhousie*
(née Olding)

1897
Laura Armstrong *Trinity*
Katharine Bruce *Toronto*
(née Bradshaw)
Kate Buck *Trinity*
Harriet Cockburn *Trinity*
(née McMillan)
Anna McFee *Trinity*
Adelaide Turner *Queen's*
Jean Willson *Toronto*

Katherine Lorigan *Bishop's*
Jessie Macdonald *Bishop's*
Martha Shaw *Dalhousie*
(née Brown)

1898   Jean Bailey *Toronto*
(née Cruikshank)
Jessie Birnie *Trinity*
Margaret Blair Gordon
             Trinity
Margaret Gould *Trinity*
Florence Harrison *Western*
Anna Henry *Trinity*
Elizabeth Scott Matheson
             Trinity
Margaret Wallace *Trinity*

Minnie Gomery *Bishop's*
Susannah Marion Hansford *Bishop's*
Lavinia McPhee-Green *Manitoba*

1899   Margaret Best *Trinity*
Margaret Fraser *Trinity*
Minerva Greenaway *Trinity*
Janet Hall *Trinity*
Rowena Douglas Hume
Trinity
Annie Macrae *Trinity*
Dorothea Orr *Trinity*
(née Johnston)
Annie Schilstra *Trinity*
(née McConnell)

Mary Morris *Dalhousie*
(née Randall)

1900   Caroline Brown *Trinity*
Mary Crawford *Trinity*
Eleanor Elliot *Trinity*
(née Edwards)
Susanna Grant *Trinity*
(née McCalla)
Mabel Hannington *Trinity*
& *Toronto*
Margaret Johnston *Trinity*
(née McCallum)
Helen MacMurchy *Toronto*
Belle Oliver *Trinity* &
Toronto

Mary Bird *Bishop's*
(née Runnells)
Margaret Currie *Bishop's*
Victoria Ernst *Dalhousie*
Winifred Reynolds
(née Braine) *Dalhousie*

1901   Annie Lapp *Trinity*
Minnie McDonald *Trinity*
Isabella Mitchell *Trinity*
(née Little)
Margaret Parks *Trinity*
Martha Smith *Trinity*
(née Doyle)

Florence Piers *Dalhousie*
(née O'Donnell)

1902　Emma Connor *Toronto*　　　　Martha Bradshaw *Dalhousie*
　　　Isabella Davidson *Trinity*　　　(née Philp)
　　　(née Thomson)
　　　Annie Davis *Trinity*
　　　Kate McLaren *Toronto*
　　　Elizabeth McMaster *Trinity*
　　　Mabel Mortimer *Trinity*
　　　(née Cassidy)
　　　Annie Ross *Trinity*
　　　Electra Wilson *Toronto*
　　　(née Anderson)
　　　Isabella Wood *Trinity*

1903　Eleanor Bennet *Trinity*　　　　Minna Austen *Dalhousie*
　　　(née Lucas)　　　　　　　　　Grace Rice *Dalhousie*
　　　Mary Bryson *Trinity*
　　　M. Jean Haslam *Toronto*
　　　(née Hoyles)
　　　Lucy Patterson *Trinity*
　　　Olive Wease *Trinity*
　　　(née Rea)

1904　Jessie Allyn *Trinity*　　　　　Blanche Crawford *Dalhousie*
　　　Dorothea Brown *Trinity*　　　(née Munro)
　　　Lucetta Morden *Trinity*　　　Eliza Mackenzie *Dalhousie*
　　　E. Victoria Silverthorn　　　Jemima Mackenzie *Dalhousie*
　　　Queen's (née Reid)　　　　　Stella Pearson *Dalhousie*
　　　　　　　　　　　　　　　　(née Messenger)

1905　Elizabeth Bagshaw *Toronto*　　Mary Smith *Dalhousie*
　　　Georgina Crawford *Trinity*　　(née Mackenzie)
　　　(née Urquhart)
　　　M. Ellen Douglass *Trinity*
　　　Lilian Langstaff *Toronto*
　　　Edith Liddy *Toronto*
　　　(née Beatty)
　　　Margaret McAlpine *Toronto*
　　　Jessie McBean *Toronto*
　　　Mary McCarthy *Toronto*
　　　(née Callaghan)
　　　Hanna Reid *Toronto*
　　　Minerva Reid *Toronto*

NOTE: *In cases where a person has received more than one medical degree, only the date of the first is given here.*

APPENDIX III
Women Graduates in Medicine in Canada 1906-1923

1906 Alice Baxter *Toronto*
Mary Campbell *Toronto*
Mary Cornish *Toronto*
(née Beattie)
Edith Hooper *Toronto*
(née Weeks)
Melissa Manderson *Toronto*
Cora Palmer *Toronto*
(née Murdoch)
Annie Sanford *Dalhousie*
(née Hennigar)
Lily Taylor *Toronto*
Rachel Todd *Toronto*
Ah Mae Wong *Toronto*

1907 Margaret Calder *Toronto*
Laura Hamilton *Toronto*
P. Jane Manson *Toronto*
(née Sproule)
Maud L. Menten *Toronto*

1908 Mary Lee Edward *Toronto*
F. Evelyn Leacock *Toronto*
(née Windsor)
Rosamond Leacock *Toronto*
Sara McVean *Toronto*
Estelle Smith *Toronto*

1909 Lily Mathieson *Toronto*
(née Boyington)
Millicent Morden *Toronto*
Jennie Robertson *Toronto*
(née Smillie)
Bessie Singer *Toronto*
(née Pullan)

1910 Edna Guest *Toronto*
Bessie Houston *Dalhousie*
(née Bober)
Jessie McDonald *Toronto*
Minnie Spencer *Dalhousie*
Catherine Woodhouse *Toronto*

1911 Eliza Brison *Dalhousie*
Stella Cunningham *Toronto*
Elizabeth Davis *Dalhousie*
(née Balcolm)
Susie Fotheringham *Toronto*
Isabella Roberts *Toronto*
Elizabeth Stewart *Toronto*
M. Agatha Wyatt *Toronto*
(née Doherty)

1912 Ethel Hayes *Toronto*
Geraldine Oakley *Toronto*

1913 Annabel McEwen *Toronto*
Edith Ross *Manitoba*
Jean Hunter *Dalhousie*
(née Maclean)

1914 Laura Kerridge *Toronto*
(née Moodie)
Edna Robertson *Toronto*
(née Cowling)
Ada Smith *Toronto*
(née Speers)

1915 Bessie Cathcart *Toronto*
(née Collver)
Edith Gordon *Toronto*
Elizabeth Kilpatrick *Dalhousie*
Frances McGill *Manitoba*
Isabel McTavish *Manitoba*
Hildegarde Smith *Toronto*

1916 Olive Cameron *Toronto*
(née Patterson)
Louisa Collier *Dalhousie*
(née Pennington)
Lilias MacIntyre *Toronto*
(née Cringan)
Mary Telford *Queen's*
(née Robertson)
Mazie Tryon *Toronto*
Agnes Walker *Toronto*
(née Young)

1917   Ruth Anglin *Toronto*
(née Cale)
Mary Beardmore *Toronto*
(née Becker)
Mary Johnston *Toronto*
Bertha Wilson *Toronto*

1918   Gladys Boyd *Toronto*
Mabel Bray *Toronto*
Mabelle Devins *Toronto*
(née Bulmer)
Lily Fisher *Toronto*
(née Snider)
Florence Rees *Toronto*
(née Meader)

1919   Alice Anderson *Toronto*
Sophie Granovsky *Manitoba*
Celia Jackson *Toronto*
(née Kennedy)
Marion Grant Kerr *Toronto*
Elizabeth Kitely *Toronto*
Mary Maitland *Toronto*
(née Cowan)
Lucy Marritt *Toronto*
(née Neelands)
Helen Milburn *Toronto*
(née Bell)
Florence Murray *Dalhousie*
Helen Wilson *Toronto*
(née Muir)

1920   Agnes Ann Curtin *Toronto*
Annie Dickson *Dalhousie*
(née Anderson)
Elizabeth Findlay *Manitoba*
Jessie Findlay *Manitoba*
E. Pearl Hopgood *Dalhousie*
Faustina Kelly *Toronto*
Janet Kilborn *Toronto*
(née McClure)
Florence McConney *Toronto*

1921   Isabel Ayer *Toronto*
(née Teskey)
Kathleen Bartley *Toronto*
Clara Brown *Toronto*
Esther Harrison *Toronto*
Mildred Newell *Toronto*
(née Folinsbee)

Mabel Patterson *Dalhousie*
Rebecca Price *Toronto*
Lilian Reid *Toronto*
(née Grady)
Annie Thomson *Toronto*
Alice Wells *Toronto*
(née Mooney)
May Williams *Toronto*
Margaret Wilson *Manitoba*

1922   Winifred Blampin *McGill*
Dorothy Burrows *Toronto*
Glenna Caddy *Toronto*
(née Garratt)
Lillian Chase *Toronto*
Mary Childs *McGill*
Victoria Chung *Toronto*
Minnie Cohen *Toronto*
(née Wladowsky)
Dorothy Countryman *Toronto*
(née Trapp)
Mildred Glube *Dalhousie*
(née Resnick)
Anne Laing *Dalhousie*
(née Creighton)
Mary Laughlin *Toronto*
(née Bowyer)
Lilian McDonald *McGill*
(née Irwin)
Lola McLatchie *Toronto*
Christine MacLaughlin *Dalhousie*
(née MacLeod)
Elizabeth Nesbitt *Toronto*
Eleanor Percival *McGill*
Mabel Russell *Toronto*
Jessie Scriver *McGill*
(née Boyd)
Violet Shaw *Toronto*
Florence Stark *Toronto*
(née Speers)
Marian Templin *Toronto*
Elizabeth Thurrott *Dalhousie*
Mary Tom *Toronto*
Grace Vanaturo *Dalhousie*
(née Cragg)
Ada Wallace *Manitoba*
(née Wilson)
Angelini Wregerinik *Manitoba*

1923 Grace Baker *Toronto*
Anne Batshaw *McGill*
Phyllis Black *Toronto*
(née Young)
Ellen Blatchford *Toronto*
(née Comisky)
Marie Cameron *Manitoba*
Ida Carpenter *Toronto*
(née Oke)
Margaret Collins *Dalhousie*
(née Chase)
Sara Cook *Toronto*
Gladys Cunningham *Manitoba*
(née Story)
Emma Gibbons *McGill*
Nora Gillis *McGill*

Dora Harie *Toronto*
(née Adams)
Flora Little *Toronto*
(née Gauld)
Hollie McKinnon *Toronto*
(née McCormick)
A. Doris Monypenny *Toronto*
Florence Pipon *Toronto*
(née Macdonald)
Gertrude Rhodes *Toronto*
Ethel Robertson *Toronto*
Pearl Rose *Toronto*
(née Summerfeldt)
Frances Schlitz *McGill*
Phebe Thompson *Dalhousie*
(née Christianson)

NOTE: *In cases where a person has received more than one medical degree, only the date of the first is given here.*

APPENDIX IV
Women Graduates in Medicine in Canada 1924-1973

UNIVERSITY	1924 to 1928	1929 to 1933	1934 to 1938	1939 to 1943	1944 to 1948	1949 to 1953	1954 to 1958	1959 to 1963	1964 to 1968	1969 to 1973	TOTAL
Alberta	5	5	8	15	14	18	16	10	33	69	193
British Columbia							20	25	24	40	109
Calgary										3	3
Dalhousie	10		4	1	3	10	14	15	25	36	118
Laval				4	11	10	20	30	31	87	193
Manitoba	18	16	21	21	21	28	20	13	24	30	212
McGill	11	15	8	31	35	37	29	42	52	74	334
McMaster										7	7
Montreal					12	24	36	37	79	101	289
Newfoundland										4	4
Ottawa						4	10	25	36	50	125
Queen's					2	16	18	20	30	52	138
Saskatchewan							9	13	22	20	64
Sherbrooke										33	33
Toronto	46	56	41	55	61	84	68	79	95	172	757
Western Ontario	2	13	11	13	14	18	18	20	31	56	196
TOTAL	92	105	93	140	173	249	278	329	482	834	2775

SELECTED BIBLIOGRAPHY

Abbott, Maude E.S., 'Autobiographical Sketch,' 1928. *McGill Medical Journal* 28: 127-152, Montreal, 1959
— Maude E.S., 'Women in Medicine'. *University Magazine,* McGill, Montreal, 1911
Albemarle, Lord, *Fifty Years of My Life.* London, 1876
American Medical Association, *American Medical Directory.* Chicago, 1923
Barr, Pat, *To China with Love; The Lives and Times of Protestant Missionaries in China, 1860-1900.* Secker and Warburg, London, 1972
Bell, E. Moberley, *Storming the Citadel; The Rise of the Woman Doctor.* Constable, London, 1953
Berton, Pierre, *The National Dream.* McClelland and Stewart, Toronto, 1970
Buck, Ruth Matheson, 'The Mathesons of Saskatchewan Diocese'. *Saskatchewan History,* 8: 53-62, Saskatoon, 1960
— Ruth Matheson, 'Making of a Doctor'. *Century 1867/1967,* Southam Press, February 13, 1967
Burwash, Nathanael, *History of Victoria College.* Victoria College Press, Toronto, 1927
Cameron, Airdrie, *Dr Charlotte Whitehead Ross.* Unpublished paper in Provincial Archives of Manitoba, Winnipeg
Clarke, Flora, *Sisters; Canada and India.* Maritime Press, Moncton, 1939
Cleverdon, Catherine Lyle, *The Woman Suffrage Movement in Canada.* University of Toronto Press, Toronto, 1950
Edwards, David, *Notabilities of Toronto.* Peter A. Gross, Toronto, 1877
Federation of Medical Women of Canada, unpublished *Minutes.* Federation Archives, Ottawa
Galbraith, John S., *The Hudson's Bay Company as an Imperial Factor, 1821-1869.* University of Toronto Press, Toronto, 1957
Gleichen United Church Women, *The Gleichen Call. A History of Gleichen and Surrounding Areas 1877 to 1968.* Gleichen, 1968

Gooderham, G.H., *Doctors to the Indians Whom I Have Known.* Unpublished
   manuscript in Glenbow-Alberta Institute, Calgary
Gray, James H., *Red Lights on the Prairies.* Macmillan, Toronto, 1971
Gullen, F.C., *Gullen History.* Manuscript scrapbook in Victoria University
   Archives, Toronto
Hedin, Sven, *Through Asia.* Methuen, London, 1898
Hilliard, Marion, *A Woman Doctor Looks at Love and Life.* Doubleday,
   Toronto, 1957
— Marion, *Women and Fatigue: A Woman Doctor's Answer.* Doubleday,
   New York, 1960
House, Canon John, *Old Sun Anglican Residential School, Gleichen, Alberta.*
   1933
Innes, Mary Quayle, ed., *The Clear Spirit; Twenty Canadian Women and
   their Times.* University of Toronto Press, Toronto, 1966
Jackson, Mary Percy, *On the Last Frontier; Pioneering in the Peace River
   Block.* Toronto, 1933
Jamieson, Heber C., *Early Medicine in Alberta; The First Seventy-five Years.*
   Canadian Medical Association, Alberta Division, Edmonton, 1947
Kilborn, Omar L., *Heal the Sick; An Appeal for Medical Missions in China.*
   Missionary Society of the Methodist Church, Toronto, 1910
Lovejoy, Esther Pohl, *Women Doctors of the World.* Macmillan, New York,
   1957
MacDermot, Hugh E., *One Hundred Years of Medicine in Canada (1867-1967).*
   McClelland and Stewart, Toronto, 1967
— Hugh E., *Maude Abbott; A Memoir.* Macmillan, Toronto, 1941
McGuigan, Dorothy G., *A Dangerous Experiment; 100 Years of Women at the
   University of Michigan.* Center for Continuing Education of Women,
   Ann Arbor, 1970
MacMurchy, Helen, *Infant Mortality; Special Report.* L. K. Cameron,
   Toronto, 1910-12
— Helen, *Sterilization? Birth Control? A Book for Family Welfare and Safety.*
   Macmillan, Toronto, 1934
— Helen, *The Almosts; A Study of the Feeble Minded.* Houghton Mifflin,
   Boston, 1920
Medical Women's International Association, *Bulletin,* Jubilee Number, 1970
Middleton, Dorothy, *Victorian Lady Travellers.* Routledge and Kegan Paul,
   London, 1965
Mitchell, Ross, *Medicine in Manitoba; The Story of Its Beginnings.* Winnipeg,
   1954
Morgan, Henry, J., ed., *The Canadian Men and Women of the Time; A
   Handbook of Canadian Biography.* Toronto, 1st edn. 1898, 2nd edn. 1912
National Council of Women of Canada, *Women of Canada; Their Life and
   Work.* 1900
Nicholson, Mary Anna, *100 Years of Medicine, 1849-1949.* Modern Press,
   Saskatoon, 1949
Orchard, Rev. Malcolm L. and Miss K.S. McLaurin, *The Enterprise; The*

Jubilee Story of the Canadian Baptist Mission in India, 1874-1924.
Canadian Baptist Foreign Mission Board, Toronto 1924

Rae, Isobel, *The Strange Story of Dr James Barry.* Longmans, London, 1958

Reid, Helen Evans, *All Silent, All Damned.* Toronto, Ryerson, 1969

Ridley, Hilda, *A Synopsis of Woman Suffrage in Canada.* Undated booklet, Stowe Collection, Victoria University Archives

Rijnhart, Susie Carson, *With the Tibetans in Tent and Temple.* Fleming H. Revell Co., 1901

Robinson, Marion O., *Give My Heart; The Dr Marion Hilliard Story.* Doubleday, New York, 1964

Scriver, Jessie Boyd, 'McGill's First Women Medical Students'. *McGill Medical Journal* 237-243, 1947

Smith-Shortt, Elizabeth, Unpublished diary and letters, Adam Shortt Collection, Queen's University Archives, Kingston

Statutes of Ontario, Queen's Printer, Toronto, 1865-1869

Stewart, Elizabeth L., *A Brief History of the Women's College Hospital.* Toronto, 1956

The Methodist Church of Canada, *Our West China Mission.* Missionary Society of the Methodist Church, The Young People's Forward Movement For Missions, Toronto, 1920

The Missionary Society of the Church of England in Canada, *Kangra Interlude.* Toronto 1946

The Women's Missionary Society, *The Story of Our Missions.* The Women's Missionary Society of the Presbyterian Church in Canada, Toronto, 1915

Thompson, Joanne Emily, *The Influence of Dr Emily Howard Stowe on the Woman Suffrage Movement in Canada.* Unpublished Thesis, Wilfrid Laurier University, Waterloo

Trout, William H., *Trout Family History.* Meyer-Rotier Printing Co., Milwaukee, 1916

Walsh, James J., *History of Medicine in New York; Three Centuries of Medical Progress.* National American Society, New York, 1919

JOURNALS

Alumnae News, Queen's University
Canada Lancet, Toronto
Canadian Medical Association Journal, Toronto and Ottawa
Canadian Nurse, Montreal and Ottawa
Canadian Practitioner, Toronto
Christian Guardian, Toronto
Historical Bulletin of the Calgary Associate Clinic, Calgary
Maritime Medical News, Halifax
McGill Medical Journal, Montreal
Montreal Medical Journal, Montreal
Nova Scotia Medical Bulletin, Halifax
Queen's College Journal, Kingston
RCMP Quarterly, Ottawa
Revue Médicale du Canada, Montreal
Western Canada Medical Journal, Winnipeg

INDEX